PRAISE FOR COLLABORATIVE HELF
FRAMEWORK FOR HOME-BAS

"I really like how the authors point out that a strengths-based approach does not necessarily have to be cliché. This is an important message to the field and cannot be stated enough. This book is great at showing how being strengths-based can be real and useful to supporting change in people. Also, it provides the reader with a clear understanding of why the collaborative helping approach is important and how to implement the approach. The vignettes and examples are excellent! I see this book as a teaching tool and I would use it in a course geared for future helping professionals. It provides useful information that encourages helpers and the organizations in which they work to be more people-centered."

Mario Hernandez, PhD
Professor and Chair
Department of Child and Family Studies
College of Behavioral and Community Sciences
University of South Florida

"This book will be helpful for those who struggle with establishing, developing, planning, and motivating clients, as it offers many examples and solutions for helping those clients most difficult to reach and engage in the treatment process. Reading this book will enrich practice methods for many in the helping professions."

Richard J. Gabriel, LCSW
Manager BHS Social Work

"The often polarized and fraught relationship of front line mental health and social service workers and the pained and troubled families with whom they work is at last replaced with one capable of generating hope, resiliencies, and lasting change. Madsen's original Collaborative Therapy Model is vibrantly transformed here—a living tapestry weaving multiple complex theories into an accessible practice shaped by the sheer humanity of care-givers and care-receivers in the most dire circumstances. From students and brand new human service workers to long experienced therapists, supervisors, and program directors—all must read this book. Hold tight to the stories within; as they fill your head, your heart, and your imagination, you will do more compassionate and effective work with those you meet next."

Evan Imber-Black, PhD
Professor and Program Director
Marriage and Family Therapy
Mercy College

"Respect and regard for people served resonates throughout, and helpers reading this book will feel understood and encouraged. Influences from Narrative therapy, Wraparound, and Motivational Interviewing are intelligently integrated in the framework, guiding service providers, supervisors, and consultants to put connection, curiosity, and hope into practice. The text addresses sensitive issues, difficult dilemmas, complicated scenarios, and serious matters in pragmatic and empathic ways, showing 'collaborative inquiry,' 'contact before content' and 'connection before correction' in action."

Marisol Muñoz-Kiehne, PhD
Clinical Psychologist, Associate Director of Training
Marin County Mental Health and Substance Use Services
San Rafael, CA

"Madsen and Gillespie have drawn strategically from cutting edge material from family therapy, as well as community and organizational development, to promote collaborative ways of working with individuals and families. Tempered by their practice wisdom and management experience, the book includes a wide range of clinical strategies that can be applied immediately by new and very experienced practitioners. Their writing truly is grounded in a spirit of respect, connection, curiosity and hope."

Peter J. Pecora, PhD
Casey Family Programs and the University of Washington

"*Collaborative Helping* is a major contribution to helping relationships of all kinds; personal and professional. Drawing on many years of experience as professional helpers, the authors offer a comprehensive set of practical and wise principles that inform the creation of collaborative, compassionate, and empowering helping relationships in a way that is both useful and inspiring. I found this book to be immediately relevant and useful in my own work as a psychotherapist and supervisor and I highly recommend it to all who are interested in improving their capacity to help others."

Andrew Tatarsky, PhD
President, Division on Addiction
New York State Psychological Association
Director, the Center for Optimal Living

Collaborative Helping

A Strengths Framework
for Home-Based Services

WILLIAM C. MADSEN
AND KEVIN GILLESPIE

WILEY

Library of Congress Cataloging-in-Publication Data:

Madsen, William C., 1954–
    Collaborative helping : a strengths framework for home-based services/William C. Madsen, Kevin Gillespie.
        pages   cm
    Includes bibliographical references and index.
    ISBN 978-1-118-56763-0 (pbk. : alk. paper)
    ISBN 978-1-118-74645-5 (ebk.)
    ISBN 978-1-118-74649-3 (ebk.)
        1. Home care services.   2. Home nursing.   I. Title.
    RA645.3.M335   2014
    362.14—dc23
                                                            2013045087

Printed in the United States of America
V10016437_121819

Contents

Acknowledgments   vii
Introduction   xi
About the Authors   xix

CHAPTER 1   **Helping: What, How, and Why**   1
             Stories of Helping Relationships   1
             Walking and Talking   8
             Helping Activities—The *What* of Helping   9
             Relational Connection—The *How* of Helping   12
             Experience and Stories—The *Why* of Helping   14
             Placing Collaborative Helping in a Broader Context   17
             Moving Collaborative Helping Into the Future   20

CHAPTER 2   **Cornerstones of Collaborative Helping**   23
             Collaborative Helping as a Principle-Based Approach   23
             Collaborative Helping and Relational Stance   26
             Collaborative Helping and a Focus on Life Stories   33
             Collaborative Helping and Inquiry   40
             The Cornerstones in Plain English   46

CHAPTER 3   **A Map to Guide Helping Efforts**   49
             Introducing Collaborative Helping Maps   50
             The Collaborative Helping Map in Action   52
             Organizing Vision and Preferred Directions in Life   53
             Obstacles and Supports   58
             The Plan   64
             The Usefulness of a Map   68

CHAPTER 4   **Collaborative Helping Maps in Different Contexts** 69
             Using Collaborative Helping Maps in Residential Programs   69
             Using Collaborative Helping Maps to Enhance Conversations
                in Child Protective Services   78
             Using Collaborative Helping Maps in the Changing World
                of Health Care   91
             Current and Potential Uses for Collaborative Helping Maps   96

CHAPTER 5   **Engaging People to Envision New Lives**   **99**
Engagement—Who Are You and What Is Important to You?   99
Vision—Where Would You Like to Be Headed in Your Life?   102
Engagement Difficulties   108
Engaging a Youth With a No Problem Stance   111
Engaging a Woman With a No Control Stance   115
Difficulties Developing a Vision   118
Connecting to Build Desired Futures   123

CHAPTER 6   **Rethinking Problems and Strengths**   **125**
Rethinking Strengths and Needs   126
Conversations About Problems as Obstacles Separate from People   127
A Map for Externalizing Conversations About Problems   135
Conversations About Strengths as Intentional Practices of Living   139
A Map for Conversations About Strengths   142
Applications of Conversations About Strengths   144
New Conversations About Problems and Strengths   148

CHAPTER 7   **Dilemmas in Home and Community Services**   **151**
Concrete Help, Boundaries, and the Terrain of Home
   and Community Work   152
The Contribution of Family Partners to Collaborative Helping   159
Relational Stance and Advocacy Efforts   161
Power Dynamics in Working With the Larger Helping System   162
Dilemmas in Advocacy Efforts   166
Helping People More Effectively Advocate for Themselves   173
In the End, It's Still Walking and Talking   174

CHAPTER 8   **Sustainable Helping**   **177**
Using Collaborative Helping Maps to Enhance Supervision   177
Building Institutional Structures That Support Collaboration   183
Building Organizational Cultures That Support Collaboration   190
A Brief Look Back   199

References   **203**
Index   **209**

Acknowledgments

There are so many people, organizations, and communities that deserve our thanks and recognition that it's hard to know where to begin. So we'll start with the people who told us such wonderful stories of helping relationships over the course of 5 years. You are truly amazing and we will always hold you close to our hearts. We have learned so much from you, and you have inspired us with your commitment, creativity, and passion. There were a number of people whose stories may not have found their way into this book but whose contributions to our own personal and professional growth have been considerable nonetheless. We hope that everyone we talked with in the course of writing this book knows that you have taught us much and that we are grateful for those lessons. Some people shared expanded stories of their work and we want to single them out for special acknowledgment. They include Rebecca Brigham, Marianne Diaz, Lindsay Legebokoff, Shaheer Mustafa, Karley Trauzzi, John Yakielashek, Anthony Irsfeld and the incredible family partners at Worcester Communities of Care, Yolanda Coentro (who was director at the time) and the staff of Safe at Home at the Home for Little Wanderers, Thomas Conley, Beth Strassman, and other staff members of Integrated Services of Appalachian Ohio, Beth Root and workers at Scott County Human Services, Charyti Reiter and the staff at On the Rise, staff members at the Carson Center and Fresh Start for Families, and the various agencies involved with the Gang Reduction and Youth Development (GRYD) Program in Los Angeles County. Other workers and family members generously gave their time and asked that their names and identifying information be changed. While you aren't mentioned by name here, please know that your contributions are greatly appreciated.

We are indebted to the many scholars and deep thinkers throughout the varied learning communities of therapy, child welfare, social service, and health care. Our work builds on your strong foundation of intellectual curiosity and creativity. While there are many different sources that have influenced us in our work, we particularly want to acknowledge narrative and solution-focused approaches, appreciative inquiry, motivational interviewing, signs of safety, wraparound, and multisystemic therapy.

There is an old African phrase, "It takes a village to raise a child." We think the same holds true for "raising a book" and want to thank a number of people without whom this book would not have come of age. We want to thank Rachel Livesy, our editor at Wiley for her continual support throughout this project. We would also like to thank the following external reviewers who read and extensively commented on the draft manuscript—Aileen Cheshire, DipEd, Unitec Institute of Technology, Auckland, New Zealand; Richard J. Gabriel, LCSW, Cadence Health BHS Social Work Services, Illinois; Mario Hernandez, PhD, University of South Florida, Tampa, Florida; Evan Imber-Black, PhD, Ackerman Institute for the Family, New York, New York; Marisol Muñoz-Kiehne, PhD, Marin County Mental Health and Substance Use Services, Novato, California; Benjamin M. Ogles, PhD, Brigham Young University, Provo, Utah; and Naomi Chedd, Licensed Mental Health Counselor and Educational Consultant, Lexington, Massachusetts. Your comments helped refine the manuscript into a much better book.

Bill would like to particularly acknowledge and thank Silvana Castaneda, Vicki Dickerson, Anthony Irsfeld, Shaheer Mustafa, Beth Root, and John Vogel for their generous and generative comments on significant or entire portions of the unfolding manuscript for this book. I would like to thank Kevin for inviting me on this journey and David Epston for urging me to take it on. It has been a life changing enterprise. Finally, I'd like to express my very deep appreciation for my partner in love and life, Meg Bond. You have both endured and supported my immersion in this project and have consistently offered profoundly useful conceptual and editorial comments. This book, along with my life, is much richer for your presence.

Kevin would like to offer special thanks to Integrated Services of Appalachian Ohio for allowing us to set up shop initially and for continued support over the years. Enormous thanks to Bill for opening up worlds I only vaguely understood, at first, as a possibility. And as a nurse by profession, I'd also like to acknowledge the special cultural memory and tenacity of strong working women and men throughout all the health and human service fields. Over the years I have witnessed extraordinary vision by everyday helpers too numerous to mention here. They often seem to be holding our world together by sheer force of intuitive helping. But the most personal kind of thanks is reserved for the strongest woman I know, Terri Gillespie. My lifetime partner is a creative, accomplished helper and my best critic. Her presence is felt throughout the book.

Finally, we want to acknowledge and thank the many individuals, families, and communities we have encountered over our combined 60 years of work. You are truly the ones who have taught us the most about doing this work. In the midst of service systems that aspire to be helpful but all too often fall short, we deeply appreciate your grace and generosity in continuing to help us learn more about Collaborative Helping. We dedicate this book to you and hope that it contributes in some small part to a way of helping that we can hold with pride.

Introduction

Welcome! We are glad you are reading this book and hope that it will support you in your work and/or studies. This book is about helping people. It is applicable for anyone with the intention to be helpful to others, including people from the many disciplines that work within the broad context of health and human services. However, the people we have had most in mind while writing this book are case managers, outreach workers, family support workers, child welfare workers, home health care workers, and residential workers. We want to particularly honor and acknowledge this vast army of people who are in the trenches of frontline home- and community-based work. We hope that this book provides easily accessible and immediately applicable descriptions of ways to approach helping work that is likely to become increasingly important in an environment of health-care reform. In this introduction, we begin by sharing how this book came to be, where the ideas came from, and what brought us to write it.

How We Came Together

We met for the first time several years ago at a neighborhood café in Cambridge, Massachusetts, over lunch. From that time on, we have engaged in an extended process of exploring, reasoning together, and, at times, even bickering about the nature and structure of a practical framework for helping that can be used across the full range of health and human services. We have been on this journey together for more than 5 years.

Bill is a family therapist with many years of training, consultation, and coaching under his belt related to the development of service models that put families at the center of strength-based, culturally responsive services. Bill's work takes him to wherever forward-thinking agencies aspire to put families and communities first. Kevin is a nurse with "hands on" management responsibilities for an emerging health and human service organization that addresses behavioral health, permanent supportive housing, employment, and, recently, integrated primary health care.

Kevin initially approached Bill with an immediate need for consultation for his agency but also with a vague idea for a book about helping that would build upon Bill's prior publications, including *Collaborative Therapy with Multi-Stressed Families* (1999, 2007a). The idea was to begin by piloting ideas together in the rural Appalachian hill region of Ohio where Kevin works every day and then move across the nation and around the world collecting and creating a patchwork quilt of stories from helpers and those they serve. As an experienced trainer, Bill was able to collect most of the stories since his work takes him all over the world. As an agency executive director, Kevin brought an important focus on the ever-changing forces of health and human services systems. Together, we have written this book. Writing as a team is not easy, but we trust that your reading of our work will provide straightforward evidence of the benefits of a collaborative approach.

INFLUENCES ON THE DEVELOPMENT OF THIS BOOK

This book is based on information from three main sources. Most immediately, we have reflected on our own experiences of doing this work. Between the two of us, we have more than 60 years of experience in health and human services where we have sought to promote collaborative ways of working with individuals and families. Over our careers, we have done frontline work, provided supervision, developed and administered innovative programs, and conducted training and consultation both nationally and internationally. A second source has been writings by others that we have found inspiring and sustaining. This book draws from cutting edge material from family therapy, community and organizational development, and post-modern thinking, always with an eye toward incorporating ideas and practices that promote more respectful and responsive ways of interacting with individuals, families, and communities. Finally, and perhaps most important, preparation for this book has involved extensive interviews with skilled frontline workers as well as individuals and families seeking help. Initially, we asked workers, "For you, what is at the heart of effective helping? Concretely, what does that look like on the ground in everyday practice? What challenges do you run into in helping relationships? How do you respond to those challenges? What might be some lessons from your experience for our field?" We also asked people receiving help about their experiences with helping (both positive and negative), how they thought our field could get better at being helpful, and what they thought would be most important to consider in that process. As the book took shape, numerous workers began to put the ideas into practice. So, we decided to seek out stories of how they were applying these ideas in order to learn from those experiences. Additionally, as we encountered supervisors and managers who were excited by these ideas, we collected stories about how they found ways to support and sustain the collaborative spirit of this work in their leadership roles. Collectively, these stories have shaped our thinking, enriched our own lives, and appear throughout this book. Hopefully, they bring to life a framework to help us find a way forward through the ambiguous, uncertain, and complex challenges of home and community work.

WHY WE'RE WRITING THIS BOOK

Authors write books for many different reasons with various hopes, purposes, and intentions. Here are two quick stories that begin to capture some of what has brought each of us to this effort.

Kevin's Story

My own story of helping starts as a hospital nurse. As a young man, I worked mostly in large academic medical centers, at first in critical care cardiology then in hematology/oncology units. There were many specialists and lots of experts. The intense learning was exciting with a pace and energy related to heroic lifesaving technical medicine that was, in a way, seductive. The teamwork of young doctors and nurses working among renowned physicians in a high pressure environment was something to remember. But for me, there was something missing. Our stance with "patients" was too often far from collaborative. Treatment options emanated from a distant professional perspective and were directed into a vacuum of communications. The complexity of personal and family affairs was almost always overwhelmed with the one-way force of medical imperatives. Life and death decisions were reduced to a shallow science intended to extend physical existence, even for a short time, with little regard for the subtlety of life well lived.

I had a dilemma. Although there was much I enjoyed in the atmosphere of the academic medical center, I wanted something more for my life's work. I didn't know it at the time, but I was looking for a more collaborative way of helping. So I returned to graduate school to prepare as a health administrator with a fairly clear plan to work my way up the chain of academic medical center nursing administration but also with a goal of helping to change the way people and families participate in end of life decision making. But then as life would have it, things changed. Long story short, while at graduate school I also married, connected with the green hills of Appalachia and was recruited by a visionary behavioral health administrator who had accepted a formidable challenge. He was charged with converting a regional psychiatric state hospital to build a community-based system of care for youth with serious behavioral disorders. We were able to obtain federal support to move fairly quickly and we used part of the venture funds to create the service organization I have led for nearly 20 years. By now we do many different things. We still serve youth and families in partnership with public child welfare agencies and juvenile courts. But we also develop and provide services for permanent supportive housing for people and families who are homeless. And we are on the frontline of integrating behavioral health with primary care as we broaden our scope to include entire communities with a new focus on issues like aging and the years, months, and weeks at the end of life. So as you can see, my journey has come full circle to be thinking now about an entire life well lived. But all along the way, my own story has always been about a more collaborative way of helping.

Bill's Story

I have a strong conviction that at its core this work is about how we are with people. Much of my life's work in this field has been about finding and developing helping practices that assist workers (and myself) to ground our work in a spirit of respect, connection, curiosity, and hope. After I wrote the first and second editions of *Collaborative Therapy with Multi-Stressed Families*, there were a number of people who thanked me for writing the book. They often said some variation of "Your book resonated for me. It had some great ideas about doing this work. But most important, it lent credence to things that I value in this work and it was great to see that in print." That has been deeply gratifying. However, more poignantly, there were also people who shook their heads and said, "I'd never read that book. Collaborative Therapy? I'm not a therapist, I don't do that therapisty stuff!" (even though their work was profoundly therapeutic). I found that sad and troubling— particularly since other people in similar jobs were among the folks who found the book so supportive. In my heart, I am a practitioner and even though I spend a lot of time providing training and consultation, I approach the work from the perspective of a practitioner. I have spent much of my professional life straddling the down and dirty world of frontline practice, where collaboration is not some esoteric idea but a basic survival strategy, and the rarified world of complex ideas that are extremely useful but often expressed in an almost incomprehensible fashion. I think these worlds of lived and learned knowledge have much to offer each other and have sought ways to bring them together into mutual dialogue. When Kevin approached me with the idea of developing a practical framework for helping across a wide range of contexts, it struck me as an opportunity both to expand the process of helping beyond a narrow "clinical" realm and perhaps tweak the class system of professional helping in which credentials often trump experience. We have sought to write a book that marries wisdom from the daily experience of doing this work in extremely challenging situations with a framework that can help workers from across the spectrum step back, reflect on your work, and try on some new ideas and practices that hopefully can support you in the work.

Overview of the Book

Chapter 1 begins with three stories of helping interactions to both jump right into the work and set a context for examining common helping activities, highlighting the central importance of relationship, and suggesting the usefulness of realizing that we all organize our lives into stories and that those stories shape our sense of identity or "who we are." With this in mind, helpers can approach people with a particular focus on the kinds of life stories we might be encouraging in our interactions with them. This chapter sets the context for the remainder of the book.

Chapter 2 presents four core concepts that serve as the foundation for Collaborative Helping. In an era of manuals and protocols, it highlights the usefulness of a principle-based approach to work that is inherently messy. It further examines ideas about relational connection and a story metaphor that were introduced in Chapter 1. And it introduces the power of inquiry (the process of asking thoughtful and compelling questions) as a crucial helping skill.

Chapters 3 and 4 outline a simple map to organize helping efforts and show applications of this map in different contexts. Chapter 3 introduces a map to help people develop a vision of preferred directions in life, identify obstacles to and supports for that vision, and develop a concrete plan to draw on supports to address obstacles to get to that vision. An example of work by a home-based outreach worker with a family provides an illustration to explore the areas of this map in detail. Chapter 4 examines ways in which helpers in residential, child protective services, and home health care have applied these maps in their work to both help them think their way through complex situations and provide a structure for useful conversations about difficult and challenging issues.

Chapters 5 and 6 move from an overall approach to helping to a more particular focus on the actual conversations that happen between helpers and the people they serve. Chapter 5 outlines concrete ways to engage people in helping efforts and help them develop visions for their lives moving forward. It places particular emphasis on ways to accomplish this combined process in challenging situations. Chapter 6 offers some novel ways to think about problems and strengths and provides guidelines to mix practical help with purposeful conversations that minimize shame and blame and maximize engagement and participation.

Chapter 7 highlights some of the dilemmas that arise when working in people's natural environments. Traditional notions about "boundaries" take on a very different cast in outreach contexts and this chapter offers a number of thoughts on those dilemmas. It also offers concrete tips for effectively advocating for people served while remaining connected to the broader helping system.

Chapter 8 explores ways to sustain collaborative work, promote systems change, and build institutional supports for a different approach to helping through specific supervisory, management, and organizational practices. It features stories from managers who have developed innovative ways to build organizational cultures that encourage respect, connection, curiosity, and hope within their organizations and brings together the previous material in the book with a focus on efforts to sustain Collaborative Helping.

Over the course of this book, we intend to move back and forth between stories of everyday helping and reflections on a framework that can guide frontline workers in their efforts to be helpful. We hope the framework provides a larger organizing focus and the "stories from the field" highlight particular ways to put these broader ideas into practice. With this in mind, let's get started.

About the Authors

William Madsen, PhD, Founder and Director of the Family-Centered Services Project.

Bill provides international training and consultation regarding collaborative work with families. He assists community and government agencies develop institutional practices and organizational cultures that support family-centered practice. Bill has spent his professional life straddling the down and dirty world of frontline, public sector practice and the exciting but more esoteric world of family therapy theorizing. He has developed and currently consults with numerous innovative home-based programs. He has written numerous articles and is the author of *Collaborative Therapy with Multi-Stressed Families* (2nd edition). In 2013, Bill was awarded the American Family Therapy Academy's Distinguished Contribution Award for Family Therapy Theory and Practice for work largely related to this book.

Kevin Gillespie, RN, MHSA, Executive Director, Integrated Services of Appalachian Ohio.

Kevin has many years of experience combining direct service, system development, and administrative management, mostly throughout the Appalachian region of Ohio. He is a registered nurse with much of his work focused on creating collaborative solutions with partners across health and human service systems and in alliance with therapeutic, housing, and employment professionals. Related to his responsibilities as Executive Director of Integrated Services and through recent involvement with an array of health-care reform ventures, Kevin is exploring themes of social innovation to reframe a sustainable local network approach to build home and community dimensions for person-centered health homes. All of his consulting, teaching, and system design work is grounded in a deep appreciation for the ageless cultural knowledge associated with everyday helping.

CHAPTER 1

Helping: What, How, and Why

STORIES OF HELPING RELATIONSHIPS

Helping relationships sustain people, they provide support in times of joy and crisis, and they strengthen families and contribute to a sense of community. The desire to be helpful may run deep across cultures and different walks of life, but the skills of helping do not always come easily or naturally. This book describes a principled framework intended to assist anyone who wants to make intentional helping a part of his or her life. We call the framework Collaborative Helping. This chapter begins with three stories of helping relationships and uses them to examine the what, how, and why of helping. The *what* is the content of helping activities (What are we doing?). The *how* refers to the process of helping endeavors (How are we doing what we're doing?). And the *why* reflects the overall purpose of helping efforts (Why are we doing what we're doing?).

Henry's Story as Told by a Helper[1]

I worked with a poor White family with four kids in foster care. Henry, the single father, had beaten one of the boys with an electric cord, and the kids were about to be placed in permanent custody of the state. No one had been able to make any progress with the family. Henry was very suspicious and had refused to meet with Child Protective Services (CPS). He'd had problems with the courts on and off for years and many workers were scared of him. Lots of them knew him by name and made jokes about his family, calling them all "losers" and being convinced they'd never change. The family was referred to us as a kind of last-ditch effort before CPS removed the kids.

So, after several attempts, I got in to see Henry, and he was skeptical and very slow to trust anybody. I tried to find something to connect with him on and he told me he grew up in eastern Tennessee. Well, I grew up in eastern Tennessee, and we learn we're from the same small town. So, that gave me a little inside track with him, but he was still pretty hesitant about working with me. After a few more visits, he finally began to open up a bit. He said "I got all these letters from CPS and I don't know what they are." So, he brought out a shoebox full of letters from CPS and admitted to me that he couldn't read. He had never told anybody that he couldn't read. Since he wouldn't meet with CPS, they kept sending him letters with the case plan and what he needed to do. And, because he couldn't read, he just put them in a box and didn't follow through. Well, we went through the letters and I explained to him what all he needed to do in order to meet the plan for reunification. The kids were kind of mixed on what they wanted, but the whole family agreed to work on the plan that had been spelled out.

Henry doesn't drive, so I would pick him up, take him to both his drug counseling and random drug testing appointments and he never missed one. Now, our county is very weak with their drug testing and it probably would not be admissible in court. You pee in a cup and they stick a piece of cardboard in it and if it turns blue then it's positive. Well, one time, the girl who was reading the drug test said, "I don't know. Kinda looks positive but I'm not sure." And when she filled out the form she marked it positive and I told her, "This man is trying to get his children back and you are sending the court a document that you are not sure about. That's not fair. You have to be sure in what you're saying." Well, my taking up for him made major points, and from then on Henry began to trust me a bit more.

In the meantime, we worked with the kids and the court allowed supervised visits, and they went well and that changed the CPS worker's opinion of Henry. The thing is, nobody understood his culture. He grew up in the back country of eastern Tennessee where when kids misbehaved, you roughed them up. I'm not saying that's right, he definitely went over the line, but that's all he knew. As we went on, people began to see a man they had never seen before. He was very sincere and serious about making sure the kids knew how much he loved them and that he didn't want to hurt them. Well, the kids began to look forward to the visitations and before long the kids all agreed that they wanted to go back with Henry. So, it came down to court time and the judge was pretty prejudiced against him and determined not to let the kids go back home. But, everybody else involved went into court and threw so many positive things at the judge that he had no choice but to say, "Okay, let's give it a try." That was 3 months ago. Now, the kids are back home and things are going well. We're still in the home providing follow-up services to the family. Henry has been very cooperative; the kids are in school and doing pretty good.

That's a remarkable story. What would you say helped to make this happen?

Well, I think I got beyond all the preconceived notions about this family. People saw Henry as a loser and didn't understand why he wasn't going along with them. Nobody had discovered that he couldn't read. And, it wasn't that he wasn't willing to be compliant. There was a pride issue there. He didn't want to admit to these people that he couldn't read. But once the barrier was broken down and a bridge was built, he was finally willing to admit, "I can't read." When he understood what they were asking of him, he was willing to go along with it because it made sense to him.

And how did you build that bridge that allowed something different to happen?

Well, I knew his culture and he felt comfortable knowing I knew where he came from. And I wasn't judgmental like a lot of the other people from agencies that had been in there. You know so many agencies come across with this attitude of "I'm here, you gotta jump through my hoops, and you can't do anything about that." And, I try to go in with the approach of "I'm here, but I'm not here to hammer you or to pass judgment on you. I'm here to help you if you want and if I can." You've got to earn the right for people to trust you and be willing to work with you.

And what are some of the ways in which you go about earning that right?

Identify a common ground. There's always common ground. Any time you walk into a home, you can look around and find something to connect around. And once you find that common ground, you can build a relationship around that, and that's going to open doors that will help them let the walls down.

Amira's Story as Told by Her

I live in a rat trap apartment in the city with my three kids. I haven't seen their father in years and figure he's either in prison or dead. My mother lives upstairs and goes back and forth between hounding me to make a better life for my kids and complaining that I think I'm better than her. I probably drink more than I should, but other people seem a lot more worried about it than me, so I've had a number of professionals parade in and out of my life for way too long. So, two of my kids were having trouble getting to school and I got "informed" that I'm going to get some help for that. I wasn't too keen on this, but said, "Okay, whatever. . ." I figured I could bluff my way out of this like I had done with everything else. So anyway, one morning this worker comes to my apartment. I was in a bad mood. It was hot, our fan was busted, the kids were whining, and the fact that I was hung over probably didn't help either. Anyways, there was just this din in my head and someone is banging on the door 'cause my frickin' landlord won't fix the bell. And, I had forgotten about the appointment and was thinking "Who the hell is that and what do they want?" and I open the door and here's this worker who looks like she's 12. I remember our appointment and I'm embarrassed and ashamed standing there in my bathrobe and without thinking, I snap, "Who the 'F' are you and what are you doing in my hallway? Get the hell out of here!" And she smiles sweetly and says, "I'm sorry I caught you at a bad time. Would it be better if I came back tomorrow?" I slam the door in her effing face. Anyway, she leaves a card with a note and sure enough next morning, she's there knocking on my door again. And she keeps doing it. She's like the Energizer Bunny—she just keeps going and going and going. And, finally, I let her in and find out she's not that bad to talk to.

What convinced you she was not that bad to talk to?

Well, first of all, she was direct and honest, no beating around the bush like that usual sickeningly sweet and smug, "How can we help you, Ms. Jackson?" when they already have their answers to that question. She started out telling me what in particular the people at school were worried about with my kids and why she was coming to my home. Then she took time to get to know me and learn about what I was worried about. She also asked me about what was working well and seemed to be even more interested in that. And she was really curious, she seemed to enjoy talking with me and I kind of liked talking to her.

So, it sounds like things got off to a good start. What happened afterward that was important to you?

Well, a few things. I felt like we were in this together. When she asked me questions, it felt like we were exploring things together rather than her grilling me with a clipboard. The plan we came up with came from both of us and made a lot more sense to me. In the past, people had come in saying, "You got to do this, you got to do that." And I'm thinking, "WTF? I'm looking for a job to support my family and that's a full-time job. I'm raising three kids and that's a full-time job and now I've got to go to all these appointments and that's a job and a half. Where am I gonna find time to do 3½ jobs?" And she came along and said, "How can I help with all you got on your plate? I can't do it for you, but I'm glad to do it with you." And I was like, "My Lord, finally someone who's on my side." And I was much more willing to take the extra time to meet with her. The other thing she did was continually ask, "How is this going for you? What are we doing that's working and what could we do that would be more helpful? And she really meant it, you know? She was really interested in whether what we were doing was useful to me. That was pretty crazy!"

That's cool! Was there anything else she did that was particularly helpful from your perspective?

Yeah, she was the first worker I've had that acknowledged she was White. Like I'm Black, in case you didn't notice, and I've had a hard time of it being Black and I don't raise that with White workers, which is most of what I've had, because I worry they'll think I'm just "playing the race card" and so I just sit on that stuff and pretend it's not there and end up seething. And when she introduced race into our conversations, I thought "Wow, that's one crazy White woman. Maybe she gets this and maybe I can really talk to her." It kind of told me that I could trust her and I could talk about stuff that was important to me.

So, how did she introduce race into the conversation and what was it about how she did it that was important to you?

Well, sort of what I said to you, she said, in case you haven't noticed it, I'm White. We both laughed and she went on to tell me that she was pretty comfortable working and living across color, but realized she still had a lot to learn and wasn't sure whether me being Black and her being White would be a problem, or no problem, or kind of a problem, and she just wanted to put it out on the table so it'd be there to talk about if that made sense. But you know, I don't think it's just about race. It's like us folks that you all are trying to help, we live in a really different world than you do and you come into our world and pretend to be all good meaning, like you're contributing to some charity for Christmas, and you got to realize how annoying that is. We don't need charity, we need help, we need someone who is willing to step into our life and stand with us. Just because we're having a hard time traveling doesn't mean we're incapable of traveling. It just means it's hard and she really got that. She didn't hold herself above me and seemed like a normal person and when she wasn't "all that," I didn't have to be "all not that." And that's the crux of it for me. She didn't judge me and that allowed me to talk more openly to her about stuff I normally don't tell you folks.

Amanda's Story as Told by a Helper

I worked with a White woman living out in the country in a trailer. When I got the referral, they said, "You can't go out alone. This woman is homicidal, schizoaffective, and off her meds." So, two of us went out and we were both pretty nervous. It's out in the middle of nowhere, down a little dirt road with no cell service and no neighbors and so if she was in fact homicidal and decided she was going to hurt either of us, we would have really been in trouble. So we went in and she had her guard up and you could tell that she was a tough cookie. She had been a stripper, she had been on drugs, she had been raped as a child and had her childhood taken away from her, and she had run the gamut and had no reason to trust anyone. What brought her to us was she had been a truck driver and had hurt herself and wanted so badly to rejoin the workforce again.

So, we went out for the initial meeting where we were supposed to do an assessment to find out what was going on in order to develop a plan to help her. Well, we went out and enjoyed meeting her. And, we ended up just talking and listening to her for a long time, and by the end of that first meeting, we realized that despite what we had been told, she wasn't homicidal. She was just pissed with the way things turned around in her life and now she's sitting in the middle of our county on welfare, receiving in a month a fourth of what she got in a week in her job as a truck driver. She was just crushed. And through working with her over a year she began to regain some sense of hope in her life. We just clicked and her guard came down.

How did that happen? What was your contribution to her guard going down?

I listened and I shared with her some of the things I've gone through in my life to help her understand where I'm coming from and help her believe that I might be able to understand what she's telling me and that I can understand that it's not just her, it's not just that she's bad people. Systems help us sometimes and systems hurt us sometimes and it's a matter of understanding that and picking out where we're going to let systems help or hurt us. Sharing those kinds of things helps people to believe that perhaps we can "get" their experience. And once she started to trust me, we talked and it helped her figure out what she wanted and how she might get there. And now, her case is closed. She went back to school, became an LPN and got a job, got married and is very happy in her life out of state. She called and invited me to come down for Thanksgiving and I said, "No, I can't do that, but I appreciate the offer." And I'm so happy for her and thinking about this just makes my heart feel so great.

These are incredible changes you're describing. What would you say might have been your contribution to these changes?

I believed in her and helped her believe in herself. She had been stepped on and kicked around and crushed and told she couldn't do anything and she's nuts and she's crazy and she shouldn't go off her meds because she's going to kill somebody and she's a terrible mom, and I just saw her in a very different light. I told her, "Okay, you've gone through all this. That's in the past. We can make it better now by going to the community college and getting your life back on track." And she said, "No, I can't do that." And I said, "Sure you can, I'll go with you to register." I think this work is about opening up doors for people. We have the key with our resources and we need to use them to stand with people and help them gain respect, success, and self-sufficiency. It took a while, but she finally had people in her life that weren't there to judge and give consequences, but were there to listen. We have the ability in our job to accompany people on their journeys. A scary journey can be not so scary if you have someone walking with you. We can help start the process when people have no sense of how to begin and they then pick up and build on it. It's empowering to have someone say, "We can do this. It might be a little scary, but we'll get through it." Amanda later told me that at the time she borrowed my belief in her to believe in herself. I thought that was really powerful.

WALKING AND TALKING

These stories are rich. There is much to learn from them even without extra analysis. Nonetheless, let's take a moment to pull out a few important themes. These three helping workers are not traditional "therapists" though we would argue that their work is profoundly therapeutic. At the same time, they are not simply "case managers." That phrase does not do justice to the complexity that goes into their work. There has been a historical distinction between "therapy" and "case management" or "concrete services." We want to suggest a new way of thinking about this work. Historically, talk therapy has consisted of a series of scheduled appointments where patients or clients come to a clinic or office to talk with a therapist who is considered to be an expert.[2] A common approach has been to provide a compassionate space where people can express themselves, work through issues, and develop insight into inner conflicts. We'll refer to this as "sitting and talking." If done well, there is no doubt that talk therapy can be life changing. Supportive services or case management, on the other hand, is most often seen as a process where helpers link people with services and provide practical assistance to get the daily work of life done. Helpers are frequently cautioned not to become "junior therapists" And yet home-based, community-centered work is strongly influenced by the dominant themes of traditional therapy. Helping efforts are often divided into these two categories of doing therapy or providing case management. We want to suggest a new way of thinking about Collaborative Helping that introduces the idea of *walking and talking*. By this, we mean stepping into a person's everyday life to engage in conversations over time while also assisting with routine needs, helping to solve problems, and taking on life's vexing dilemmas together. If you are already doing this kind of work, you know what we mean. Practical helping combined with purposeful conversation can work best when it is organized around the stories that shape people's experience of their lives. This approach draws on a narrative metaphor that has become increasingly popular in our culture and focuses on the stories that people tell about their lives and that organize how they make sense of their lives. Within this frame, the work is not about sitting and talking with people to work through their issues but walking and talking alongside them in ways that open up opportunities for them to experience themselves differently and change their life stories. The new possibilities that this process can open up are potentially quite powerful.

HELPING ACTIVITIES—THE *WHAT* OF HELPING

What are some of the helping activities that workers are doing in each of these three stories? First and foremost, they are engaging people by "meeting them where they are." While the injunction to "meet people where they are" is a common one in the helping profession, it may be a bit more difficult to do in actual practice. Henry, Amira, and Amanda had developed reputations that made it challenging to work with them for good reasons. They could each be very difficult to work with and they had provoked a number of troublesome reactions from many different helpers. It's important not to minimize these challenges and engage in some politically correct "Oh, aren't they resourceful" kind of thinking. A commitment to looking beyond initial reputations, taking time to get to know people outside their immediate difficulties, and earning the right to serve them when they are behaving badly can be quite a challenge. It may require helpers to bite their tongues, hold back their initial inclinations, and think carefully about how they might best respond. Engagement and the process of building relationship is not simply an initial step before we get down to the "real" work of helping. It is the heart of our work that both directs and is nourished by the work itself. It needs to be attended to always. We will come back to the importance of relational connection repeatedly.

A second activity that is routine and in most instances required of helping workers is to formally assess a person's status in order to develop a plan to move toward some safer, better, and/or healthier future. This is usually accomplished through some sort of assessment followed by a written service plan. The ways these efforts are undertaken have clear and lasting effects on people served. The assessment and service plan activities in the earlier stories focused on resourcefulness and were done in collaboration. For example, Amira commented that assessment questions felt to her like a joint exploration and described the plan that emerged as making sense to her since it was created together. Active involvement of people and families in assessing and planning for their own lives contributes to a sense of influence, encourages ongoing participation, and is more effective and efficient. As another mother we interviewed put it,

> I think it would make a big difference if parents who are having
> a difficult time could have more input into their service plans.

And if you had more input into the service plan, how would you respond differently to the service plan?

> I'd be motivated to do it faster because I would figure it would
> work. I'd get things I needed for me and my family and, in doing
> that, I'd probably be more open to what others were asking of
> me. I think the motivation to do the service plan is directly cor-
> related to how much input I have into making that service plan.

A third activity described in our stories is of workers engaging in concrete efforts to help people make desired changes in their lives. This is at the heart of walking and talking. Some of these efforts involved working directly with people, like monitoring Henry's supervised visits with his children and helping other family members to take steps toward reunification. Others involved linking people and families to additional community resources and following along as partners to determine practical usefulness. Often, linkage with services and supports involves serving as translator between people, families, and others in the community. Henry's story recalls his helping worker literally reading and translating the written material sent from CPS and stored away in Henry's private shoebox. Sometimes focused advocacy is called for, like Henry's worker calling out the woman who did the random drug testing or Amanda's worker helping her walk through the registration process at the community college. We often are needed to walk alongside the people we serve. We do not walk in front, nor behind, but together along the way.

A fourth activity that is alluded to but never directly identified in the stories shared so far is hearing, holding, and bearing witness to people's own story. This may well be the most important helping activity of all. As another group of workers in an outreach home-based program put it,

> We go out and hear the stories no one wants to endure. The fact that we listen to these stories, bear witness to them, and acknowledge and validate the people telling them is a huge part of our job that has never been captured in our official job description. We listen to the stories no one else will hear. But the important thing is not *that* we listen, but *how* we listen. We listen to validate their pain and simultaneously acknowledge their resilience – the "keep on keeping on" of everyday life. That resilience gets lost in the crap of daily problems and our job is to remember it, keep it alive, and honor it.

People served often describe a sense of feeling like they are being repeatedly judged and criticized by workers and programs originally designed to serve them. They also recognize the power of being heard and feeling acknowledged. It is crucial that the importance of this does not get lost in the business of our helping work.

To summarize, we have identified the following activities of effective helping:

- Engaging people and families with genuine respect.
- Using assessment as a "two-way introduction" to establish connection and to further build relationship through collaborative planning.
- Actively helping people to make practical changes in their lives through services with a focus on what works, and translating and advocating for people.
- Hearing, holding, and bearing witness to people's own stories.

In descriptions of each of these activities, we have also touched on the ways the activities are undertaken. We think the *process* of service delivery is inseparable from the *content* of service delivery and want to emphasize the importance of not just focusing on *what* help is offered, but *how* that help is offered.

RELATIONAL CONNECTION—THE *How* OF HELPING

To set the stage for this discussion, let's examine a continuum of ways to define helping. A dictionary definition of *helping* is pretty simple— "an act or instance of giving aid" (*Webster's 3rd New World International Dictionary*, 2002). However, the same dictionary definition of *help* is more complex with many nuances. Here are some of them:

- To cooperate, assist, or support
- To be of use to or further the advancement of
- To give aid; be of service or advantage
- To remedy, stop, or prevent
- To succor or save

Each of these definitions places people who are helping and people who are being helped in different kinds of relationships with each other, ranging from a very hierarchical relationship of being "remedied, stopped, or saved" to a more lateral relationship of "cooperating, assisting, or supporting." We know there are times that may call for swift decisive action, like life threatening or otherwise extremely dangerous situations. But in general, we are proposing a spirit of helping that leans more toward the "cooperate, assist, support" end of this helping continuum. We think a more collaborative approach reflects how people generally prefer to be treated and as a result tends to be more effective. The way a helping relationship is defined has powerful effects on the experiences of those receiving help. It affects how they experience themselves in the helping process, it affects how they experience the helping relationship, and it affects their beliefs about the possibility of change. Helping efforts that contribute to a sense of competence, connection, and hope are both more humane and more effective.

Collaborative Helping invites workers to shift from a relational stance of an "expert" repairing dysfunction to an "ally" assisting people to envision and move toward a more desired life with attention to everyday issues like health, family, work, and a place to live. Bill has previously described the central importance of the attitude that helpers hold, including the usefulness of a relational stance of an appreciative ally where people experience workers as "in their corner, on their side, or standing in solidarity against problems in their lives." (Madsen, 2007a, p. 22). Some of the cross-cutting themes in the earlier stories help to illustrate this kind of relational stance.

One emergent theme is *respect*, characterized by humility, trust, and accountability. Helpers in the earlier stories carry immense respect for the people they serve. Henry's worker shows humility in describing the importance of "earning the right" to come into Henry's life rather than assuming it as part of a job description. Amanda's worker describes the importance of telling stories from her own life to gain trust and to help Amanda believe that she might be able to understand her situation. Amira describes her worker's continued commitment to getting feedback on how their work together is going in order to learn what is useful and what is not. She demonstrates a commitment to make helping accountable to Amira as the person who is in the best position to make an intelligent judgment about what is helpful.

Another important theme is *connection*. Henry's worker emphasizes the importance of finding common ground and building bridges. Amira describes how her helper acknowledged differences between them as a basis to build on similarities saying, "She was the first worker who acknowledged racial differences between us." Amanda's worker and Amira both highlight the importance of engaging others as "regular folks." Amanda's worker talked about efforts to tell stories that put her alongside rather than above Amanda while also acknowledging that the people we serve are usually in a more vulnerable position. Amira commented that when her worker was not "all that," she was freed up from being "all not that."

The next important theme for effective helping is *curiosity*. This involves some critical reflections on our own preconceptions to deliberately step into the life experience of another person including a broad appreciation of the larger context. Amanda's worker describes the importance of seeing beyond a mostly negative picture of Amanda presented in the initial referral. Henry's worker describes the pervasive stereotypes held by the professional community about Henry's family and the usefulness of getting to know Henry and his family beyond initial stereotypes. Amira talks about the importance of her worker understanding the stress of demands for multiple appointments. The process of stepping into another person's experience requires suspending our own preconceptions. We must acknowledge limits in our ability to transcend stereotypes as the first step toward doing just that. Curiosity means that we also cultivate a larger appreciation of family, community, and culture. Amira's worker acknowledged the potential impact of racial differences on their work together, while Amanda's worker acknowledged that "systems sometimes help us and systems sometimes hurt us."

A fourth theme for helping is one of enduring *hope*. Amanda's worker described believing in her and helping her believe in herself. Belief in people's resourcefulness and the possibility of change is not simply an idea or a feeling. Instead, it is a commitment put into everyday practice. Amanda's worker walked with her into the community college registrar's office and Henry's worker took him to random drug tests and non-naively believed in the possibility of his sobriety. As we move beyond simple themes of helping, we'll be sure to look more into some actual practices of hope. We'll explore some of the ways gifted helpers "do" hope. For now, let's just say that the practice of hope is reflected in a combination of appreciating the challenge of hard traveling and believing that people served have what it takes to travel a hard road.

There are many ways we can approach people in our work. Helping relationships are a two-way street so we can't ignore the contribution to that relationship of the people being served. But workers do hold a special leadership role. As helpers, we have choices about the attitude or relational stance we take and how we respond to the different ways people interact with us. We can develop practices that help us to stay grounded in respect, connection, curiosity, and hope, even when strong forces and our own emotional responses pull us toward judgment, disapproval, and disconnection. The attitudes we hold, the relational stance we take, and the way we position ourselves with the people we serve all have powerful effects. The next section develops our thinking about a story metaphor to further explore these ideas.

EXPERIENCE AND STORIES—THE *WHY* OF HELPING

We have examined both the *what* (content) and the *how* (process) of helping. Now let's take a look at the *why* (purpose) of helping relationships. Obviously there are many different purposes that organize our interactions with the people we serve. However, we think a focus on the stories that define people's lives can guide us in a most extraordinary way. Henry, Amira, and Amanda's stories are not simply stories that are told. They are also stories that are lived. In the process of interacting with others, we all experience ourselves in particular ways. These experiences shape our sense of self and identity. The stories we tell about our lives determine the range of possibilities that are available to us. Here is a brief story that illustrates this from Margie, a woman who has sought many different kinds of help over the years.

> I used to have this wizard of a therapist who I met with multiple times a week for many years. He was brilliant and I probably wouldn't be alive today if it wasn't for him. I felt like he did great work, given the material he had to work with (me). After our meetings, I would come out aware of how broken I was and how lucky I was to have him to help me. More recently, I've been meeting with my outreach worker and she's pretty good; not as smart as that therapist, but I have to say it has never occurred to me when I walk away from those meetings that I'm broken. I come away feeling strong and confident and believe I can take on my life and that feeling has been incredibly helpful.

Margie experiences herself in very different ways in her interactions with the therapist and the outreach worker.[3] While she talked about similar issues with both helpers, she came away from one feeling broken and from the other feeling strong and confident. We will examine the usefulness of a story metaphor for our work in more depth as we progress. For now, we simply observe that people experience their sense of self in the context of relationships. Interactions with helpers have the potential to shape the stories that enable people to make sense out of life. A simple saying from a popular postcard highlights this shift in thinking.

> *Life isn't about finding yourself. Life is about creating yourself.*

> —Unknown

Identity is not fixed. Instead, identity is something that evolves and changes in the course of interacting with others and telling the stories of our lives. This way of thinking about identity shifts helping efforts from searching to *find* Margie's essential self (is she broken or strong and confident?) to interacting with her in ways that help to *create* or bring forward preferred stories and related experiences of self. In this instance, her experience with the second helper invited an experience for Margie of feeling stronger and more confident. A focus on the stories that shape people's lives combined with awareness of how helping interactions affect those stories means that every interaction is a unique opportunity that holds the promise of inviting experiences of self in ways that can open up or close down possibilities. Margie's experience of herself as strong and confident is likely to carry her further in her life than an experience of self as broken and in need of repair. The next story from an employment support worker captures the application of this kind of experience to our work.

> I think respect and courtesy are at the heart of my work. A lot of people we deal with are often not treated with respectful courtesy and that relates to their self-esteem and that relates to their employability, even though in a roundabout way.

Can you say more about that?

> Yeah, sometimes we perceive ourselves by the way we're perceived by others and I think that if you treat somebody with courtesy and respect like they deserve it, they may see themselves differently and we need our consumers to see themselves differently if they're going to change. I see myself as a merchant of hope and a lot of my job is selling a new idea or a new identity.[4] The biggest problem that I see for many of the people we work with is how they think about themselves—"I'm a loser and I'm just gonna roll in that because that's who I am and it's all I can be." And I see my role as giving them opportunities to expand that and treat them differently because maybe they will then see themselves differently and have an experience of how it feels to be treated with courtesy and help them come to believe that they are worthy of courtesy and that then others are worthy of courtesy and it's a whole different way of being in the world. I refuse to play along with that old story and try to treat people in ways that they see opportunities to succeed and do what other people do and have what they have.

What do you think it might mean for them to have that opportunity?

> For some of them it means everything because they haven't considered having a way to live except the one they know because

that's all they've ever known. Some people may want to stay where they are, but many just don't see other possibilities and I think you can really set the wheels turning and they can play with that because that's at least a start. I think people can change; they're not stuck with their lot in life. You can reinvent yourself at any age. It may be difficult, but that doesn't mean you can't change your situation.

Helping interactions have powerful effects on how people see themselves. They shape the experience of helping and can open or close possibilities. Relational connection is both a foundation for effective helping and a powerful "intervention" in its own right. We have used stories of effective helping to identify the what, how, and why of helping. We'll conclude our initial discussion of helping by locating the Collaborative Helping framework in the broader context of other approaches and by anticipating some of the trends that may change the way we look at helping in general.

Placing Collaborative Helping in a Broader Context

Collaborative Helping is a practical, everyday framework for a wide range of helping work in homes and neighborhoods. This framework has been informed by the everyday wisdom of helpers doing this work as well as the experiences of the people who have been helped. It has also been informed by evidence-based practice and "empirical" approaches. Both sources are important and work best when combined together.

Collaborative Helping has been most influenced by well-established sources such as narrative approaches (White, 2007; White & Epston, 1990), solution-focused approaches (Berg, 1994; de Shazer, 1985, 1988), appreciative inquiry (Cooperrider, Sorensen, Whitney, & Yaeger, 2000), motivational interviewing (Miller & Rollnick, 2013), and the signs of safety approach to Child Protective Services (Turnell & Edwards, 1999).[5] These approaches provide ways of thinking and practicing that we find particularly congruent with the spirit of the work that we emphasize in this book and the specific ways in which we have drawn on them will become apparent throughout the book. Collaborative Helping fits within and is applicable to broader systemic approaches to helping such as wraparound, systems of care, and the recovery movement. It is also congruent with much of the spirit of multisystemic therapy (Henggeler,

Cunningham, Schoenwald, & Borduin, 2009) and the multisystems model (Boyd-Franklin, 1989; Boyd-Franklin & Bry, 2000). We briefly examine each of these in turn.

If you are reading this book and interested in commonsense helping as an important way of relating to people and doing your job, then it is likely you already know something about wraparound and systems of care. The very word "wraparound" has various meanings for different people across most of the helping professions. On one hand, the wraparound model has been carefully defined (Bruns & Walker, 2008; Burchard, Bruns & Burchard, 2002; Dennis & Lourie, 2006) within the systems of care movement as a collaborative team process with specific principles and practices that can be reliably implemented in a certain way. But the word is also generally used and broadly understood to describe a range of flexible approaches to health and human services that empower families and helping workers to creatively "wrap" resources and supports "around" people based on their own unique needs. Wraparound was initially developed in the 1980s as a process for maintaining youth with serious emotional and behavioral problems in their homes and communities. Over the past 30 years, policy makers, communities, and families have worked together in many instances to make systemic changes so that youth with very challenging behaviors might avoid residential treatment, psychiatric hospitalization, and in some instances, incarceration. Included among the established tenets of wraparound are many of our own ideas about ways of engaging people in a collaborative relationship.

Similarly, the mental health recovery movement, a significant trend in health and human services, views helping as a process of overcoming the negative impact of a psychiatric disability despite its continued presence with a focus on strengths and skills, hopes and desires, and connections and supports. It encourages a shift from symptom reduction to improvement in functioning, resilience, and adaptation. In 2004, the U.S. Department of Health and Human Services recommended that public mental health organizations adopt a "recovery" orientation to severe and persistent mental illness, including those dually diagnosed with mental health and substance abuse issues. Recovery-oriented models are rapidly expanding across public agencies—a development that will only continue with the rise of integrated care, a movement in which health-care teams consider all behavioral and physical health conditions at the same time with a focus on individually tailored treatment geared to the whole person. Recovery models represent a significant paradigm shift that is closely aligned with core principles of Collaborative Helping, including a focus on possibilities, collaborative partnerships, and accountability to those served. The recovery movement represents the first time a consumer-led movement has had a significant impact on mental health practices, starting a potentially radical revolution in the field. The U.S. Department of Health and Human Services (2004) has formally defined recovery as a "a journey of healing and transformation enabling a person with a mental health problem to live a meaningful life in a community of his or her choice while striving to achieve his or her full potential" (p. 2). Collaborative Helping fits very much into this vein and simultaneously seeks to broaden the focus from just mental health problems to a broader consideration of challenges that arise at individual, relational, and socio-cultural levels. As health-care reform begins to sweep through most all health and human service systems, these ideas become more valuable and relevant for more people than ever before. The essential power of the helping relationship can guide us all as we rethink a place for personal and community resilience, placing it at the heart of delivery system reform.

Multisystemic therapy (MST) and the multisystems model are current helping models often used in home and community work. MST is a focused behavioral treatment intended primarily for juvenile offender families and their communities. What MST has in common with both wraparound and Collaborative Helping is a broad holistic orientation in service planning combined with a keen emphasis on strengths. MST focuses on "finding the fit" between identified behavioral problems and the entire context of a youth's environment. It goes on to target "sequences of behavior" within and between various interacting elements in a youth's life that may maintain problems. These elements include things like family, teachers, friends, home, school, and community. Additional core elements described in MST combine to define an intensive home-based therapy intended to be carried out by a skilled practitioner under rigorous clinical supervision. MST is a highly successful behavioral intervention. But MST also shares many simple, commonsense principles of a helping relationship with both wraparound and Collaborative Helping.

The multisystemic model draws from structural and behavioral family therapy approaches. It was developed with a specific focus on poor and marginalized families and is particularly relevant as a result. It is a problem-solving approach that has generally been applied in home, school, and community settings. It takes an ecological approach, focusing on multiple levels, including extended family, non-blood kin and friends, and church, community, and helping agency resources, with close consideration of cultural, racial, and socioeconomic issues. We appreciate this focus on the broader context because the families primarily described throughout this book are profoundly impacted by poverty. The multisystemic model recognizes and addresses the real impact of the dual stressors of poverty and racism as a central part of their work. From here let's take a look at what the future may hold for our work.

MOVING COLLABORATIVE HELPING INTO THE FUTURE

Case management is too often misunderstood to be a sort of *be all and do everything to get things done* kind of service for people with complex needs. Still, because of the usefulness of practical supportive services, this kind of helping work first created for mental health has flourished, been adapted, and expanded to become vitally important across a very wide range of health and human services (Walsh, 1999). Given the immediacy of needs, the central importance of relationship is sometimes undervalued or even lost. While there may still be some room for differences of opinion about the role of supportive home and community work, surely there can be little doubt that meeting a person in his or her own home, assisting with practical needs, and engaging in purposeful conversation builds relationships and can be profoundly therapeutic.

Today, a growing legion of helpers are involved with home-based supportive helping work that builds on family and community resourcefulness. We seem to be moving rapidly toward a reformed health and human service system that goes beyond a disease treatment focus to more broadly promote health and well-being. These changes may fundamentally alter the way we think about health and wellness. Insurance and managed care companies, government payers, provider systems, and health-related professions are all engaged with policy makers to redefine how we do the work of health care to better support people of all ages and at every level of health status (Miller, Kessler, Peek, & Kallenberg, 2011). This new way of "doing" health care is often called collaborative or integrated care and is organized around patient-centered medical homes. The idea is to integrate behavioral health with primary care to create a new kind of teamwork for care coordinators, health coaches, and home health workers on an expanded health-care team that, of course, still puts physicians and nurses right in the middle of the action. It's not really that different from supportive services we have known in the past. Emerging trends seem to point toward a more holistic way of thinking about how people, families, and communities rely on practical helping to remain well. In the United States alone a modest estimate that cuts across professions predicts that up to one million people will be doing some kind of home-based, community-centered work by 2020 (Bureau of Labor Statistics, U.S. Department of Labor, 2012–2013). That number may be pushed upward as the health-care industry discovers what mental health already knows. Practical and supportive home and community-centered services can help people and families achieve their highest level of health and well-being at a relatively low cost.

Home and community workers and others who perform helping work are indispensable. They work often with very little guidance. They ask great questions, listen carefully, and have a genuine curiosity about the lives and communities of the people they serve. Out of necessity, the good ones cultivate a collaborative attitude shaped by years of working within the complexity of the natural home environment. While therapeutic models and evidence-based practices are valuable to them, home and community helping workers tend to rely more on skillful improvisation within a broad framework than on an exact script. Collaborative Helping provides just such a framework to help frontline workers focus their efforts. In the chapters that follow, we talk much more about intentional helping and outline our framework in detail. We offer many stories to illustrate real ways of practical helping. We hope our Collaborative Helping framework will assist you in moving along with your work and navigating the ever-changing currents of helping.

NOTES

1. Names and identifying data have been changed in these stories to protect confidentiality. However, throughout this book, we use the actual first names of helpers (with their permission) who have contributed through their stories.
2. A note on language—People seeking help have historically been referred to as patients, clients, or consumers. Many of the people served and the organizations that support them that we have encountered object to these labels. When asked what they would like to be called, a number of them have often replied, "Call me by my name." This may be difficult in the aggregate and so throughout this book, we will refer to people

seeking (or mandated for) help as "people." We will refer to people who are employed in helping positions as helpers or workers. We realize that helpers or workers are also people and this use of language may have marginalizing effects on them. However, it is the best label we currently have and given the choice of marginalizing people seeking help or marginalizing people offering help, we choose to risk the latter.

3. This example of a "wizard" of a therapist and a "pretty good" outreach worker who was actually much more helpful to Margie raises many issues about the class system of human services and who is more and less valued and acknowledged within that system.

4. We would question this idea of "selling" a new identity. As we'll examine in Chapter 6, we think it is more useful to think about eliciting or inviting people into new identities than selling new identities to them. We are much more interested in inviting or eliciting new experiences than in pointing out or selling new possibilities. This is a fine, but important, distinction. We'll note it now and come back to it later.

5. For readers interested in learning more about any of these approaches that have been very influential in our work, please consult the following resources: Narrative approaches (Freedman & Combs, 1996; Freeman, Epston & Lobovits, 1997; Madigan, 2010; Monk, Winslade, Crocket & Epston, 1997; Morgan, 2000; White, 2007; White & Epston, 1990; Zimmerman & Dickerson, 1996); solution-focused approaches (Berg, 1994; Berg & Kelly, 2000; Christensen, Todahl, & Barrett, 1999; de Shazer, 1985, 1988; Durrant, 1993); appreciative inquiry (Cooperrider et al., 2000; Cooperrider, Whitney & Stavros, 2008, Hammond, 1998); motivational interviewing (Miller & Rollnick, 2002; 2013); and the signs of safety approach to Child Protective Services (Turnell, 2010; Turnell & Edwards, 1999; Turnell & Essex, 2006).

CHAPTER 2

Cornerstones of
Collaborative Helping

The first chapter used stories of helping relationships as a way for you to begin to get a feel for the heart of helping. We introduced ideas about the power of relational connection and the importance of the life stories. We now follow up in more detail to describe four cornerstones that provide the foundation of the Collaborative Helping practice framework:

- It is a *principle-based* approach.
- It emphasizes the importance of the *attitude* or *relational stance* with which helpers approach individuals and families.
- It focuses on the *stories* through which people make sense of their lives.
- It emphasizes inquiry—the ability to ask meaningful and respectful questions in a spirit of genuine curiosity.

COLLABORATIVE HELPING AS A PRINCIPLE-BASED APPROACH

To get us going, consider the following story from a home-based outreach worker as an example of the complicated terrain of home and community helping work.

Heather and I got to know each other under some unusual circumstances. She was 14 years old and had been living in foster care for a while, and she had recently made the transition back home. Her family consisted of her mom, stepdad, and younger sibling. Her mother was entwined in a battle against Depression and Alcoholism. Heather had been "acting out" and had a "bad attitude," and her stepdad wasn't interested in parenting her. They agreed that Heather could meet with me for in-home counseling, but they would not participate.

At our first meeting together, Heather said she was grounded and didn't know when or how the grounding would come to an end. I helped her ask her stepdad about it given that her mom was sleeping. He said that if she did all the dishes, she could be "off grounding." They didn't have a dishwasher, so this job would have to be done by hand. I asked him if I could help her, and he said, "Sure."

We commenced our dishwashing together. Piles and piles of pots and pans and plates and cups covered the kitchen counters rendering them unrecognizable. This proved to be a gigantic undertaking. Heather was talkative, animated, full of vim and vigor. We worked for over an hour together and proudly told Heather's stepdad of our accomplishment. He walked into the kitchen, opened the oven, and said, "You're not done yet." In the oven was another huge pile of pots and pans and dishes.

I went back to see Heather the next week. She asked if we could go for a walk with Daisy. I said, "Sure!" and then asked, "Who is Daisy?" She said, "I'll show you." Heather walked upstairs and came back downstairs with a snake wrapped around her neck, and off we went for a walk.

When we arrived back to the house, the child protection worker was outside in the driveway talking to Heather's stepdad. Her mom was losing her battle with Depression and Alcoholism and had decided to go to inpatient treatment. Heather's stepdad was refusing to take care of her. The worker had come to take Heather back to foster care. Heather screamed—long and loud—ran up to her room raging and swearing. Ipods had not been invented yet. She turned on her boom box as loud as it would go. She opened her bedroom window, faced it out toward us helpers standing below, and blasted the song "I Will Survive." I thought, "I'm sure you will."

As we see from this story, decision making in home-based work rarely fits into neat all-or-none categories. Helping work is inherently messy. Workers almost always live in the "in-between." Helpers respond to surprising and unusual circumstances that often can't be anticipated ahead of time. Nigel Parton and Patrick O'Byrne (2000) suggest that any effort to force order and certainty on work that is inherently unpredictable runs the risk of entirely "missing the point." They have encouraged our field to (re)discover our traditional strengths in working with ambiguity, uncertainty, and complexity.

One way to think about rising to the challenge of working in homes and communities is what we call "disciplined improvisation." Working in a natural environment is very different from working in an office. Disciplined improvisation means responding to the messiness of everyday helping with ongoing learning within a flexible framework. We can best explain this with a story from a mother who met with Bill individually for help in dealing with her 18-year-old son who struggled with impulsivity.

> When we started, I figured I'd describe the situation to you and you'd tell me what to say to my son. However, I've come to realize that my son's impulsivity is much too clever and I will never be able to memorize all the possible lines I might need. Instead, our work has helped me to develop a role, character, or place to stand in responding to my son's impulsivity. When I'm in that role, I can respond to whatever comes at me and handle that pretty well. I want to thank you for helping me develop a place to stand rather than giving me lines to memorize.

Similarly, principle-based frameworks are an attempt to provide helping workers with a solid place to stand in responding to the messiness of this work. Home and community work is just too complicated to follow a simple recipe. The work is predictably unpredictable. Improvisation is often an inherent part of this work. But as legendary singer/songwriter Paul Simon puts it, "Improvisation is too important to be left to chance." The smooth improvisational riff of skilled jazz pianists rests firmly on top of years practicing scales and playing composed music to develop "muscle memory." Likewise, Collaborative Helping is a principle-based practice framework to support disciplined improvisation.

Meeting with people in their homes or communities often has little external structure to it. It is easy to get lost in the chaos. One way we have tried to bring structure into the inherently improvisational nature of our work is with the idea of "maps." While we live in an era of GPS systems telling us about the next move to make, we think the old-school approach of maps that help us step back from the immediacy of

the situation and get a sense of the broader terrain on which we're operating can be very useful. We return repeatedly to this idea of particular
maps that can help workers think their way through complex situations
and can provide guidance for conversations with people about challenging issues. These maps help ground workers in core values of respect,
connection, curiosity, and hope without being tied to an overly restrictive approach. These maps assist workers in developing habits of thought
and action that are the helping equivalent of muscle memory.

COLLABORATIVE HELPING AND RELATIONAL STANCE

Chapter 1 introduced the importance of attitude or relational stance
with which workers approach the people they help. Our commitment
to this issue comes from our own experiences along with lessons learned
from stories of frontline practice. But ideas about the importance of
relational stance are also supported by research from outcome studies in
psychotherapy, child welfare, and related fields. We will highlight some
of the relevant literature and then move on to show ways in which
skilled practitioners put this into practice in their everyday work.

   The common factors literature consists of 40 years of studies examining contributions to good outcomes in psychotherapy (Duncan, Miller,
Wambold, & Hubble, 2010). There is a consistent finding that 40% of
therapy outcomes are attributable to client factors, referring to what
people do in their lives outside of therapy. Thirty percent is attributable
to common factors like relationship, empathy, respect, and genuineness.
Fifteen percent is attributable to shared hope and expected change
(which we also see as a relationship factor). And, only 15% is attributable to technique, that is, what practitioners do in therapy. This literature suggests some rethinking for how we approach helping. If client
factors are the single most powerful contributor to good helping, then it
makes sense to find better ways to draw from the resourcefulness of
people and communities. If relationship and hope can be considered
together as one factor, then relational stance takes center stage. Research
on the power of the alliance reflects over a thousand findings and is one
of the best predictors of good outcomes (Duncan, Miller, & Sparks,
2004). Research from child welfare replicates these findings. Andrew
Turnell (2010) cites multiple research sources that show the best outcomes for youth and families occur when there are constructive

working relationships between workers and families and among collaborating professionals.

In the last chapter, we previewed the usefulness of a relational stance of an appreciative ally grounded in a spirit of respect, connection, curiosity, and hope (Madsen, 2007a). While these ways of being could be viewed as personality traits, we prefer to think of them as practices or ways of going about the business of helping. We might ask helpers: How do you show respect? How do you connect with people? How do you express curiosity? How do you "do" hope or otherwise bear witness to hopefulness? Seeing these ways of being as practices rather than characteristics suggests a way of helping that can be cultivated and further developed.

Holding a stance of an appreciative ally does not mean that we uncritically accept everything people say and do. It also does not limit us in taking a stand on important issues. There are times when we may decide to confront people about the effects of their actions on others and times when we may decide to act in ways that may be experienced by people as "not being on their side." Obvious examples include involuntary hospitalization or filing a required child abuse report. The important thing about taking a stand in these situations is not *whether* we do that, but *how* we do that. Respectful, open, and honest conversations about our own concerns and actions are an important part of our work. Let's also acknowledge that holding a relational stance of an appreciative ally is often easier said than done. To help accomplish this, we examine four commitments that support a relational stance of an appreciative ally and explore how frontline workers put those commitments into practice.

Striving for Cultural Curiosity and Honoring Family Wisdom

Workers and the people we serve can be seen as distinct cultures with their own idiosyncratic beliefs and ways of interacting. Helping services can be seen as a cross-cultural negotiation in which workers and people interact in an emerging relationship. We can approach each person, each family, and each community as a unique culture with a particular way of life. In doing this, we can approach each new encounter thinking of ourselves as anthropologists looking to understand the meaning of this interaction for the people we are with rather than as professionals dispensing judgment or diagnosing sickness. In this way, we take a stance of knowing very little at first as opposed to knowing almost everything as an assigned expert. A good example of this type of cultural curiosity comes from Lindsay's story about her outreach work in a remote rural community.

You've said curiosity is at the heart of your work. Can you give me an example of how you put that curiosity into practice?

> A moment that comes to mind is a woman who has had a particularly hard life. She experienced a lot of physical and sexual abuse as well as numerous addictions. This day we were talking about her addiction to heroin, which she's been clean now for 20 months. She described staying at the shelter and a new woman came in who was clearly agitated and seemed to be in withdrawal and my client described it as a trigger for her. At first, I was like, "Oh yeah, trigger. . ." But then I thought I have no idea what that means to her and so I asked her, "What do you mean by trigger? What does that mean for you?" And that question opened up a wide door of more than just what I had thought.

What did it open into?

> A lot more emotions than I had thought. So trigger to me meant that she was craving heroin, right? But it actually brought back a lot of depression and sadness. She missed her family and it brought her back to the times when she was on heroin and she began re-living all the horrible things that were going on in her life then. So it wasn't just a trigger for craving, it was trigger for a particular time in her life that she described as really hard for her.

And, in that situation, how did you make the transition from assuming you knew what she meant to being curious about what she meant? What steps did you take to make that transition? Was there anything you did in your head or anything you did before speaking to her?

> So she said trigger and I said, "Oh, yeah." (Like I have any idea of what it's like to come off of heroin.) And I thought of supervision and the emphasis we constantly have on touching base with people and asking what does that mean for you. And I thought I'd better check in with her and see what that meant to her. So I asked, "What does a trigger mean for you? Like, this is what it means for me, but I have no idea what it is for you, right?"

Uh huh. And, and when you asked those questions, what do you think might have been the effect on her?

> Well, like I've been saying, I don't know. But if I was in her shoes, I would feel empowered and it would open more space to trust the person I was talking with and I guess that might be true for her.

Lindsay's story describes one way of entering into people's experience and using that to build relational connection. While helping professionals have historically been encouraged to provide answers rather than ask questions, we can see from this story how curiosity builds trust and connection and can have beneficial effects on people seeking help.

Believing in Possibilities and Eliciting Resourcefulness

Let's continue to build on this cross-cultural metaphor. When we enter a different culture, what we look for profoundly shapes what we are likely to see. All families have particular competencies, know-how, and capacities to grow, learn, and change. Helping moves along more smoothly when we emphasize *what is* and *could be* rather than simply *what isn't* and *should be*. A belief in possibility does not require that we ignore or in any way minimize problems in life. But people are not their problems. In fact, viewing people as different from and more than the difficulties they face releases us to better identify assets. The importance of believing in possibilities is shown in an answer given by Karley, another outreach worker, who was asked why she thinks that belief is important.

> Well, because there has to be possibilities. If there weren't possibilities, then what would I be doing and why would people meet with me? If the way you're living your life right now is all you could ever have and if there were no other possibilities, then why would you go for any type of help? If there weren't possibilities, there'd be no need for services, or at least services that anyone could believe in.

This is a refreshing and commonsense answer. But sometimes as helpers we assume our role is to identify a problem, discover the cause, and then intervene to get people to "do the right thing." This is encouraged by documentation requirements, diagnostic manuals, and a medical model for treatment that drives most service delivery. Yet as Andrew Turnell and Steve Edwards (1999, p. 49) maintain, most assessments are too one-sided; focusing exclusive attention on deficits and dysfunction is rather like "mapping only the darkest valleys and gloomiest hollows of a particular territory." A focus on possibilities acknowledges what is going well and reveals clues about a way forward. Listen to the words of a mother talking about her helper.

> When my worker comes out to meet with me, I watch her eyes very carefully. She has these beautiful brown eyes that you could get lost in. But the thing that is most amazing is that when I look into her eyes, I see her seeing me and the me I see reflected in her eyes is the me I want to be and that gives me hope and confidence to go forward.

In this way, a focus on resourcefulness both enhances engagement and is a powerful intervention in its own right.

Working in Partnership and on Family Turf

If we believe that people often are more resourceful than we realize, our work together can become a collaborative process that draws on the know-how and abilities of both parties. This next story highlights a way in which two outreach workers inadvertently flipped the power dynamics with a family to good effect.

> So, Jeff and I go out to the family's house. And, I forget what happens, but I said something that offended the father and he says, "That's it. You're fired. Get out of here and don't come back." Well, I'm feeling really cruddy and ask him if I can use the bathroom before we leave since we have an hour drive to our next appointment. So, I go into the bathroom and do my business and flush the toilet and watch the water start rising and rising. So, I stupidly put the toilet seat down, like that's going to stop the water and then watch the water fill over the sides and run down onto the floor. Now I'm feeling like not only am I a lousy worker, but I've gone and broken their bathroom. And I go out embarrassed and tell the father and he jumps up like a man on a mission and says, "No problem," grabs his plunger and sets about fixing things. Then we go out to the car and now it's Jeff's turn to eat crow. His keys are locked in the car. Fortunately, their teenage son has some expertise in these matters and when Jeff asks the family for help, their son is Johnny on the spot with a coat hanger and quick as pie the car is open. Well, we're way

late to our next appointment and ask the family if we can use their phone since it's a rural area and there's no cell phone coverage. It's evening and Mom's cooking dinner while I call the next family to cancel our appointment and as I hang up, she says, "Hon, you've had a rough day. Would you like to stay for supper?" I'm not sure, but it smells good and so we do and we have a nice time over dinner. As we finish up and begin to head out, the father says, "So, we'll see you next week. Take care on your drive home."

What do you think happened that led to this shift?

I think in our meeting in their house the father experienced me as judgmental and superior (like I was "all that") and when Jeff and I respectively screwed up, we became regular folks and that allowed the family to become regular folks and have something to contribute and it just changed the whole dynamic between us. I think that's why they asked us back.

This shift from helpers as experts with specialized knowledge to helpers as regular folks who are journeying alongside people contributes to a partnership that validates family contributions without diminishing helpers' know-how.

Engaging in Empowering Processes and Making Our Work Accountable to People

Let's talk about a kind of empowerment that makes our work more accountable. We hear a lot about empowerment. But real empowerment means finding a way to support people in building the better life that they actually prefer. At times, even with the best intentions, helpers inadvertently constrain people's influence on and participation in their own lives. One way to avoid unintended disempowerment is by actively soliciting feedback as a matter of routine. In so doing, we become responsible partners *working with* people rather than experts *acting on* them. John is a Child Protective Services supervisor talking about accountability and the ways he makes that a priority in his work.

Accountability is important to me for building trust. For me, it's important that our office can hopefully be a place where people can get help versus the stereotypical "we're baby-snatchers," right. It's a pretty uphill battle trying to fight that reputation and yet I'm really committed to the people here in my town and want us to be seen as a group that can be trusted. And one of the ways to build trust is accountability—if I say I'm going to do something, then it's going to happen; and if it doesn't, then there's got to be a way to bring that up and hold me accountable. I think really one of the pillars of any relationship is trust and accountability.

Do you have an example of you putting that into practice?

So, there was a mom I worked with named Kalinda and we were going to court on her son. She initially brought him into care on a voluntary basis and then she didn't want him in care anymore and she wanted to pull him out and he was in a group home and we thought it was important that he actually stay there as he was making good progress. And Kalinda was developmentally a little bit lower functioning and it would have been easier to slide by and get her to sign things and there's a way in which I probably could have done that, right? But I really felt it was important that she have an advocate to make sure the process was fair. It would have been easy for me to take advantage of her and even though I thought keeping her son in residential care was the right thing, I wanted to make sure we respected and involved her in the process. So we went to court so that she could get a lawyer to represent her because I didn't feel like she truly understood what was happening in that process and I wanted her to have an outside advocate make sure the process was a fair one.

And for you, not taking the easy way out and instead moving into a process that ended up becoming more time-consuming, what does that say about what you value and care about in your work?

I think one of the very basic principles that guides me is that old adage of the Golden Rule—treat others the way you would want to be treated. And I really try to hold to that. It's important for me to pause and think "How is this for my client? If I were in their shoes, how might I feel and how would I want to be treated?"

And, if you were to offer a testimonial to other workers about the importance of accountability in CPS, what would you have to say about that?

That it is vital and that we cannot do our work without accountability. Bottom line, our work is about relationships, and relationships don't work when there's no trust. And trust requires accountability. I don't think people can move forward without a sense of accountability.

And in pressured times when it is tempting to take shortcuts, why do you think it is worthwhile to take this harder route?

In two words—job satisfaction. If you can develop a relationship with a client, that's a great thing and developing a relationship as a child protective worker is a pretty tough go. We hold a pretty big stick and the nature of that relationship is not going to be like a normal, informal relationship. Again, I'll use that analogy of walking beside someone; not dragging them forward and not pulling them back; it's like we're on this journey together.

John is absolutely right. Developing a solid connection with families as a CPS worker is a daunting undertaking. His view that constructive work requires a strong relationship, that relationships require trust, and that trust is based on accountability has a wonderful logic flow. As helpers, we are often encouraged to become *responsible for* people served. It becomes our duty to do our best to provide them with a better life. We want to emphasize the importance of being *responsible to* people served. Helping efforts, while usually grounded in good intentions, sometimes have beneficial effects and sometimes have inadvertently negative effects. The people we serve are the best judges of the effects of our actions on them; finding ways to solicit their feedback and ensure that we are accountable to them provides a foundation for the development of relational connection.

COLLABORATIVE HELPING AND A FOCUS ON LIFE STORIES

Collaborative Helping is an integrative practice framework that draws from a variety of sources. As Vicki Dickerson (2010) has pointed out, any integrative effort operates within a broader organizing metaphor that guides how we think about people, problems, and helping efforts. The Collaborative Helping framework views people's lives as being shaped by the stories they hold. Let's see how folk treasure Woody Guthrie's musings about songs might reflect on our consideration of the impact of life stories on the lives of people served.

I hate a song that makes you think that you are not any good. I hate a song that makes you think that you are just born to lose.

Bound to lose. No good to nobody. No good for nothing. Because you are too old or too young or too fat or too slim or too ugly or too this or too that. Songs that run you down or poke fun at you on account of your bad luck or hard traveling. I am out to fight those songs to my very last breath of air and my last drop of blood. I am out to sing songs that will prove to you that this is your world and that if it has hit you pretty hard and knocked you for a dozen loops, no matter what color, what size you are, how you are built, I am out to sing the songs that make you take pride in yourself.

While Woody was talking about the impact of songs people sing, we can extend this to the impact of the stories people tell about their lives. Drawing from narrative therapy ideas, we'll look at the relevance of a story metaphor in our helping work. Figure 2.1 is a pictorial representation that we'll use to start to explain this.

Imagine the dots in Figure 2.1 as the various daily experiences people go through (a good breakfast, a horrible fight getting your kids off to school, a good interaction at work, a frustrating interaction at work, a traffic jam coming home that leaves you really grumpy, a warm welcome from your partner, a tense dinner afterward, a quiet night reading alone, etc.). There are far too many events in daily life to include them all in how we might describe our day to others, or even to ourselves. So, we organize life events through stories to provide a framework for making sense of the world. A story line consists of events (the dots) in a sequence across time organized according to a theme or plot (the black line connecting some of the dots; Morgan, 2000). At any point, there are multiple stories of identity available to us and no single story can adequately

FIGURE 2.1   **EXPERIENCES AND STORYLINES**

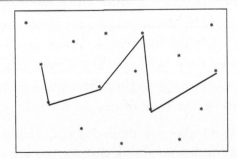

capture the broad range of all our experiences. As a result, there are always events that fall outside any single story (hence all those dots). However, over time, particular life stories are drawn upon as an organizing framework and become the dominant story that gets told about who we are, what is important to us, how we behave, and of what we are capable. These life stories make our world coherent and understandable. At the same time, in the words of Michael White and David Epston (1990, p. 11), life stories "prune from experience" those events that do not fit within them. Life stories shape our experience of life by promoting selective attention to some experiences and selective inattention to others. For example, within a story of "I have a wonderful family, but sometimes we're a little rough around the edges," you might notice certain dots in the daily list from Figure 2.1 that are in sync with this story (e.g., We had a good breakfast, getting kids to schools is often a struggle, work is work with both good and hard moments, traffic is traffic, my partner was glad to see me, it was nice to have some time to read). Within a story of "No one understands me and my home life is miserable," you might notice other dots that are consistent with this sentiment (e.g., I can't believe we had another fight getting the kids off to school, I was already pissed about that frustrating interaction at work and then I got stuck in horrible traffic on the way home, dinner was the usual mess and, once again, I ended up spending my night alone). Events that fit within the plot or theme of the dominant story are noticed and included. Those that fall outside the plot or theme are "pruned from experience."

Using a Story Metaphor to Guide Our Work

Here is a concrete example of the usefulness of a story metaphor for helping work. Fred is a large White working-class man who comes from a long line of men in the trades. He is currently unemployed due to a downturn in the economy but was previously a block mason. In his words, he is a "meat and potatoes guy who does what I want, when I want, how I want, and nobody but nobody is going to tell me different." He's recently been diagnosed with high cholesterol and his wife has been trying to interest him in a diet of tofu. You can probably imagine his response. Fred's meat and potatoes life story has little room for a medical condition that has no outward apparent signs (aside from a number on a medical report). We could view Fred as "in denial" of his medical condition. We could also view high cholesterol as something that does not fit within his organizing life story and that may be experientially nonexistent for him. In order for Fred to constructively deal with his new medical condition, he will need to not only alter his lifestyle but also his life story. The stories of our lives shape our experience of life and can enhance or limit our possibilities in responding to difficulties that develop.

At the same time, the stories that shape our lives are not simply our own. In many ways, they are received from and embedded in family of origin and broader cultural stories that organize our sense of self and our relation to the world. A continuation of Fred's story puts this in perspective. A home health worker, who worked in a program with funding flexibility that allowed him to spend a significant amount of time with people in their natural environments, was going out to meet with Fred and his wife. Fred used to be an avid hiker, but had given that up over time. The worker (also a burly White man) engaged Fred around old hiking tales and encouraged Fred to show him some of his favorite local trails (also helping Fred get the exercise recommended for him). On their walks, Fred and the worker talked about many different things, but among them was his health and diet. When asked about his objection to tofu, Fred replied, "That's girlie food. I'm not going to eat that goo." We can see how Fred's meat and potatoes life story is embedded in broader gender and class "shoulds" or expectations or specifications about what makes a "real man." In this way, individual life stories are embedded in broader cultural narratives. In talking about "manly food" and "girlie food," the worker asked Fred how his buddies might respond if he ate girlie food ("They'd tease me mercilessly"), what Fred's doctor had told him would happen if he continued eating only manly food ("I'll die right quick"), what he liked about "doing what I want, when I want, how I want" ("Being my own boss and having options"), and whether the splitting of food into manly and girlie categories gave him more options or fewer options ("You got a point there, but I still won't eat goo"). They also talked about how much Fred had been enjoying the hikes even though they were hard because he was out of shape. In the past, Fred's buddies had also teased him about hiking ("Those new age hiking stores are for Yuppies"), and Fred and his worker talked about how Fred might want to respond to that teasing in order to have more "options" as he desired. This helped Fred reconsider some of the cultural "shoulds" in his life around "girlie and manly food" and Fred decided to try some less manly food in order to get in better shape to enjoy his hiking even more. Over time, Fred continued hiking, reconnected with some of his old hiking buddies, and began to change his diet, noticing its effects on his hiking abilities. While he did not convert to the "new age tofu diet" he described his wife as trying to foist on him, he did begin to eat more chicken, salad, and fruit.

So what is the relevance of considering the broader sociocultural context to the immediate job of helping? The dominant stories in people's lives often blame them for their troubles (think of Woody Guthrie's quote on songs), portray them as unable to address those problems ("Nobody understands me and I have a miserable home life") or even "prune from experience" the existence of problems altogether (Fred and cholesterol). Considering the larger sociocultural context of individual life stories helps us appreciate the hold that particular life stories can have on people and can reduce shame and self-stigmatization. It shifts the onus of blame from the individual person to the constraining cultural ideas (Fred's wife was less frustrated when she thought about him as being caught by gendered ideas about what men should eat than when she simply saw him as a stubborn old goat). And it provides opportunities to highlight people's agency (and responsibility) in challenging those cultural expectations in order to develop and live out preferred life choices.

Helping Interactions as Definitional Ceremonies

As we highlighted in Chapter 1, interactions between helpers and the people they serve have the potential to invite people to live out or enact particular life stories. As Fred and his worker literally walked and talked, Fred reconnected to an old identity that he realized he really missed. In one of their talks, Fred commented, "I still am a guy who does what I want, when I want, how I want, but I'm getting older and if I want to keep doing all that, I've got to take care of myself." In this way, the interaction between Fred and his worker invited the enactment of a slightly different life story that opened more possibilities for constructively dealing with his medical condition. Fred had been referred to this worker because many health-care providers had been frustrated by his "denial" of his serious medical condition. Fred's worker could very likely have interacted with him in ways that would support that story of denial. If he had attempted to confront Fred with a statement along the lines of "Fred, you're in denial here and have to come to grips with the fact that you have a serious medical condition," you could imagine Fred's response. However, he interacted with Fred in a way that opened possibilities for a different life story to emerge—one of "being clear about what I want and taking care of myself to get it."

We suggest that almost every interaction between helpers and the people they serve has the potential to invite the enactment of particular life stories and so we're going to adapt another idea from narrative approaches to help us reflect on this. In Chapter 1, we highlighted a core helping activity as "hearing, holding, and bearing witness to people's stories." Narrative approaches have drawn from cultural anthropologist Barbara Meyerhoff's (1982, 1986) use of the phrase "definitional ceremonies" to develop some interesting witnessing practices (Russell & Carey, 2004; White, 1995, 2000). We will not go into the details of Meyerhoff's work here, but we want to honor the phrase definitional ceremony and extend it to a way of thinking about every interaction we as helpers have with the people we serve. Michael White (2007, p. 165) has framed definitional ceremonies as

> Rituals that acknowledge and "regrade" people's lives, in contrast
> to many rituals of contemporary culture that judge and degrade
> people's lives. In many of the degrading rituals, people's lives are
> measured against socially constructed norms, and they are judged
> to be inadequate, incompetent, disordered, and often a failure in
> terms of their identities.

While narrative approaches have used the idea of definitional ceremonies as a way to organize a formal way of bearing witness to people's stories, we think the notion of definitional ceremonies can organize our thinking about every interaction with the people we serve. Every time we meet with people, we are offering them the opportunity to live out a story that organizes their life. The ways in which we structure our interactions with them has the potential to elicit stories that will regrade and lift them up or degrade and drag them down. We think that we can intentionally organize formal and informal contacts with people as definitional ceremonies with an eye toward questions such as "How might people experience this interaction? How might they experience themselves in it? And what can we do to enhance the possibility that they will have an experience that lifts them up and carries them forward rather than drags them down?" In this way, "walking and talking" can be organized by thinking about every helping interaction as a definitional ceremony that can open possibilities for the emergence of new identities.

Here are two examples of this process in helping work. An outreach worker working with a teenager struggling with impulsivity takes him to a pool hall and teaches him how to think several shots ahead, shooting the cue ball not only with the intention of knocking a ball in but also lining up the cue ball for his next shot. He then moves to helping the boy plan, thinking two shots ahead. Rather than talking about the boy's impulsivity, he is helping him enact planfulness. A worker driving a mother to a school meeting has a conversation with her about how she would like to respond to others in the upcoming meeting, helps her think through how she might do that and see the meeting as an opportunity to enact a different way of being. On the drive back after the meeting, the worker finds ways to acknowledge how the mother was different in the meeting with a goal of supporting her in living out a different story about her life.

This idea that every interaction between helpers and the people we serve has the potential to invite the enactment of particular life stories brings home the point that every interaction is an "intervention." As a result, we need to be conscious of our "use of self" and how we interact with people at all times. This can be a sobering and perhaps scary prospect. It can also add richness and depth to our work. In this way, case management becomes more than simply "managing cases." It becomes a way to transform lives and seize opportunities to help people enact new stories of identity. With this in mind, several points become apparent. It is important to:

- Address not just presenting problems but also the broader life stories in which the problems are embedded.
- Focus on the process or the *how* as well as the content or the *what* of helping activities.
- Understand people's experiences of our interactions with them.
- Interact in ways that minimize the "living out" of constraining life stories and invite the "living out" of empowering life stories.

COLLABORATIVE HELPING AND INQUIRY

In our attempts to be helpful, we are often tempted to offer suggestions or guidance. However, simple advice is not all that helpful. Research shows its effectiveness is very limited—only 5% to 10% of people change when they are offered simple advice (Sobell, 2013). In addition, although we may have many good ideas, there are underlying dangers here. If we offer useful suggestions, we may subtly encourage a view that our presence is required for people to manage their own affairs. And if we offer bad advice, we may inadvertently convince people that their problems are so bad that even an expert can't help. Surely all helpers have found themselves at one time or another stuck in a struggle to convince someone that life would be a lot better if only they would just listen and follow our advice. Unfortunately, this can get the helper stuck in a situation that is frustrating for everyone. So we shift our understanding of helpfulness from giving advice to asking worthwhile questions. You may remember Lindsay and Karley talking about the importance of curiosity and believing in possibilities. Now they help us to think about inquiry.

Lindsay's Story of Inquiry in Action

So, you said before that for you the heart of effective helping is curiosity. What are some other ways that you bring curiosity into your work? How do you do that?

> Well, one thing I tell my clients is that I'm not an advice giver. I'm a thought explorer. That's what we're going to do together. I'll ask a lot of questions and we'll just explore your thoughts together.

That's a really interesting phrase. Can you say more about what you mean by "thought explorer"?

> Well, when I was a kid, I always kind of fancied myself a scientist or something like that. And, I've gotten a lot of feedback from clients who get put off by counselors who have said, "Well, I don't think that's a good idea. You should do this and you should do that." So, one of the things I sometimes say is, "This is not going to be a session of advice giving today. We're going to explore thoughts and just create more space for you to have room to look

at all the different thoughts." And I like that job description because it's more exciting and opens more possibilities than just setting goals and filling out forms and that kind of stuff.

And, this process of thought exploring with people, what are you hoping to accomplish with that? What's your intention here?

Just to get them thinking about their own situation or different ways they could look at it and to have a different experience as they're thinking about it. I think what's going on in someone's head when we ask them questions is where the action is and I'm hoping in the process of thought exploring that they'll have a different experience of what we're talking about.

And if you think about your preference for exploring thoughts rather than giving advice, what are the values behind that? What's important to you about that?

Well, the freedom to sort of explore your own thoughts, your own expressions, what things mean to you. The ability to knock around ideas with other people without any judgment because there's no advice or recommendation that could leave people feeling corrected or put down.

What do you think it means to other people to have you so interested in their thoughts and to have you so committed to exploring their thoughts?

Oh, I think it means a great deal. My sense is they probably feel heard and understood, and validated. I mean they keep coming back.

And, if thought exploring were more a part of our field, what do you think might be the effect on the field?

Well, not to minimize the seriousness of our work, but people would maybe take things a little bit lighter and maybe reflect more on what they're saying and doing. And there would be more validation of everyone's thoughts and I think just overall more of a relaxed sort of manner with the work.

And what effect might that have on people's experience of seeking out help?

I think people would be more open to services and not so frightened of the implications of "I'm going to see a counselor; something must be wrong with me" and move on to exploring thoughts with someone. I think we'd be really busy.

Karley's Story of the Challenges of Grounding Work in Inquiry

What are some of the challenges that come up for you in seeing your work as asking questions that open more possibilities for people?

> I don't know. Sometimes I think it could be perceived as though I don't do anything because if I'm meeting with someone who has the expectation that I might be able to fix them and I don't offer to fix them, I worry that it's not what they're expecting and they may see me as not being helpful because I'm somehow missing something or I'm being negligent or something.

And what assumptions do you think might be behind that perception?

> Perhaps their idea is that it's more about transferring my knowledge onto someone else. Like, I have knowledge and it's my job to pass it on.

And what are some of the assumptions behind your preference for asking questions?

> Well, I think probably the belief that I don't have the answers for others. I mean there's certainly some things I know, that I've learned and textbook stuff I've read. And, if people wanted to ask me about that, I could certainly help on that. But I just have this underlying belief that I don't know what would be the best for everybody. There are so many ways of coping with life and doing things, and thinking about and addressing problems and I wouldn't want to say, "Here is how you're supposed to do it."

And, as you think about your preference for asking questions to elicit people's knowledge rather than conveying your knowledge, does it seem to you that this process of asking questions is an important skill to develop?

> Yeah, 'cause it's not so easy as it seems. I mean you're not just throwing out random questions. It's very deliberate and the questions have intent to them. You know, the intent is to get people thinking or to create a different possibility for them perhaps.

And what has helped you to do this? How have you learned to ask helpful questions?

> Um, by thinking ahead, what this question might evoke or how this question might be perceived, that sort of thing. Putting

myself in the position of responding to it and thinking about how I can make it as easy as possible for people to respond and how to make it apply more to their world. For example, if it's with younger kids, how can I ask this question so that it makes sense to them?

If you were to offer thoughts or ideas to others trying to develop their capacity to ask helpful questions, what would you say?

Well, I wouldn't want to discourage people and suggest that whatever question they asked had to be a really good one. I'd say keep asking questions, just keep them coming, because somewhere in there, you'll find a good one, right? And you don't know how your questions are going to be perceived by people, but you can think about where they might take people. I'd hope the questions would be focused around exploring possibilities and creating different perspectives and making space for people to think about things differently. Not telling them how to think, but opening up space for different thoughts.

And, if you think about your job as asking questions that open up possibilities and create space for change, what do you like about that job?

I think it's interesting. It's challenging to come up with questions sometimes, but I think it's fun because you have to be creative.

And, what do you think the people you work with might appreciate about your view of your job as asking questions that open up possibilities for change?

Well, my hope would be that they would think that I'm interested and that I give a crap, you know. I think I do give a crap and I think knowing if someone gave a crap about me, that would be a good feeling, right? My experience is that people like being asked questions when you're really interested in what they're going to say. And I appreciate the connectedness that comes with this. Because in order for me to come up with questions, I have to step into their shoes and that helps me feel more connected and appreciative of the people I'm working with and that's a good job.

And, if your description of how you approach the work were a more general description of helping, what do you think it might be like for people to go get help?

I think they'd be interested, like I'll give that a try. Or, maybe weirded out because help's not supposed to be fun or counseling is not supposed to be creative from a typical view of it. But I think it would get people talking.

And, if helping was more fun and creative, how do you think that might be different for helpers?

They'd be more passionate about their work, less burnout, more possibilities for how to do the work.

There are many ways to use questions in our work. Karl Tomm (1987a, 1987b, 1988) has developed some interesting ideas about the use of different questions in different situations. He draws a distinction between *orienting questions* (questions asked about problems, behaviors, or experiences to orient the helper to the situation) and *influencing questions* (questions asked with the intention of influencing people to change their thinking, feeling, or behavior). In his consideration of influencing questions, he further distinguishes between questions that have a *corrective intent* and a *facilitative intent*. Corrective questions often contain embedded suggestions to get a person to change (e.g., Why don't you set limits on your son rather than giving in to him? If you were to use a different tone with your daughter, how do you think she might respond? Can you see that withdrawing when your partner gets upset just makes things worse?). These are essentially instructions dressed up to look like questions. The helper comes to the conclusion that something is wrong and uses questions to try to get people to change (to think, feel, or behave in more "correct" ways).

Facilitative questions do not attempt to lead or direct, but can open space for people to connect with their own resourcefulness to get to a better life of their own making. These questions might sound something like this: "When you've had problems with your son in the past, were there times when things turned out better than expected? What was different then? What was your son doing differently? What were you doing differently? What helped that to happen? What of that might be useful here?" To be sure, both corrective and facilitative questioning often hope to bring about some kind of change. But the first specifies direction while the second opens space for more self-guided change with specifics that cannot be determined by a helper ahead of time.

A corrective approach to helping is often encouraged by assumptions that promote professional expertise over family and cultural knowledge. Karley's comment that she's only seen as being productive when she's dispensing knowledge and fixing things is a good example of this pressure. However, Tomm (1988) warns that corrective questioning can position helpers in the role of judges instructing people in the error of their ways and telling them how to behave. Even when judgment is politely covert, it mostly gets in the way.

We are particularly interested in facilitative questions where helpers work alongside people. We refer to this process as *collaborative inquiry* to suggest a partnership that taps the resourcefulness of both parties. In this partnership, helpers contribute by asking facilitative questions that help people envision and develop preferred directions in life. While this is a different notion of professional expertise, we think it is an important one to claim. The ability to ask thoughtful, compelling questions that open new possibilities is an art and craft that requires detailed attention and study.

We want to suggest that compelling questions can generate powerful experiences. Let's examine what this means. If we have a strong relational connection and ask compelling, thought-provoking questions, they often generate interesting experiences. As Lindsay put it, "I think what's going on in someone's head when we ask them questions is where the action is and I'm hoping in the process of thought exploring that they'll have a different experience of what we're talking about." Here's an example of that in action. An outreach worker asks a mother, "For the past 5 years, you've had a really hard time with your son and yet somehow you've hung in there with him. How have you done that?" The mother considers this question and thinks to herself, "What is this woman talking about? I'm pulling my fricking hair out. I'm not managing this situation. Actually, we're still living together, so I guess that's managing something. How did I do that? Well, I did X and Y, but not Z. X and Y must count for something. I hadn't thought about that before. Maybe I'm doing better than I thought. Wow, that's something!" And then she responds, "I don't know." We would suggest that her internal conversation and her experience of self in that internal conversation is much more important that her eventual spoken response. In this way, the questions we ask generate an internal experience of self as people consider possible responses to those questions. With this in mind, helpers can ask facilitative questions that open space for different experiences of self to emerge. We are not trying to take people from old, bad stories to new, improved stories. Rather this is a movement from sparse, thin stories about their lives to thick, more richly developed stories. If we were to put this in terms of a soup metaphor, we could say we're interested in moving from thin consommé stories to thick stew stories.

In framing helper skill as asking compelling questions, we are not suggesting that helpers abdicate their own knowledge or values. Instead, we're suggesting that we begin by asking questions to elicit the ideas of the people we serve, then prioritize shared ideas that emerge in the conversation, and only then consider whether our own ideas might be relevant, useful, and welcome. It is important to keep our own ideas in perspective and take good care not to consider them more important than the ideas of people served. While this is a collaborative process, it is not an egalitarian partnership. The people we serve are in a much more vulnerable position in helping relationships and it is important to be mindful of the power differential that exists. In this process, helpers have particular expertise in inquiry and take on a leadership role in organizing questions while remaining accountable to people served for both the direction of that inquiry and the effects of the questioning process on them.

THE CORNERSTONES IN PLAIN ENGLISH

This chapter has covered the cornerstones that support our work. There's perhaps a danger that this comes across as abstract and highly technical. We are drawing on some complicated ideas and trying to present them in accessible ways. We don't want to dumb down this work. At the same time, many of the ideas that inform our work have historically been conveyed in some pretty inaccessible ways. So here are the four bottom lines for us.

One, Collaborative Helping is based on principles, not recipes. This work is far too complex to distill to a simple set of steps. We need to find a way to approach "disciplined improvisation" that blends a rigorous approach to our work with recognition of the inherent demands for flexible adaptation to situations we could never have anticipated. Two, Collaborative Helping is grounded in relational connection. At its heart, this work is about the attitude we hold and the way in which we position ourselves with the people we serve. Relational connection builds an important foundation for this work and can have powerful effects on the people we serve in its own right. Three, a story metaphor may sound a bit esoteric, but it's really quite simple. Every interaction we as helpers have with people affects how they experience themselves and shapes how they make sense of their life and the possibilities available to them. With that in mind, it's important for us as workers to consider the effects of our actions on the people we serve, to question what kinds of life stories our helping interactions might encourage, and to reflect on the degree to which those life stories might help or hinder them in pursuing desired lives that also have constructive effects on those around them. People often come to us as helpers because they're stuck. We want to help, but we may be more helpful by moving away from trying to provide good answers to offering thoughtful questions that help them think their way through getting "unstuck." The remainder of this book draws on these four cornerstones to set out a practical, efficient framework for helping efforts.

CHAPTER 3

A Map to Guide Helping Efforts

Chapter 1 introduced wraparound, systems of care, and the recovery movement, all of which come out of a lineage moving from family-based services to family-centered services to family-driven services. These efforts have been driven both by professional desires to provide more respectful and responsive services and by over 30 major state level lawsuits in the United States that have focused on the lack of creative service alternatives for families and the use of overly restrictive residential and institutional placements (VanDenBerg, Bruns, & Burchard, 2003). These suits have resulted in settlements promoting significant changes in service delivery in a number of states. Similar changes have occurred in health care with the development of integrated and collaborative care models.

In a study of innovative systems of care programs, Ellen Pulleyblank Coffey (2004) highlighted notable accomplishments at a macro programmatic level and raised concerns that at a micro level less attention was being paid to the actual conversations between helpers and families. She found that workers were often operating without a clear framework to guide their work, and important contributions from family therapy about engaging families, building resilience, and having helpful conversations about difficult issues were not being utilized. This chapter and the next attempt to bridge this gap by highlighting a map that can help frontline workers across many different contexts organize how they think about and talk with individuals and families in ways that keep everyday practice grounded in collaborative family-centered values and principles.

INTRODUCING COLLABORATIVE HELPING MAPS

The process of helping has historically begun with two questions: "What is the problem?" and "What caused this problem?" We could instead ask, "What might a future with fewer problems look like?" and "What gets in the way of that happening?" Often our work is framed in terms of problems that need to be addressed. There's an understandable focus on learning about the problem, what caused it, and what we might do to address it. But beginning with a focus on the problem often pulls people and helpers directly into a shared sense that life is filled with problems and little else. Instead, we can shift our initial focus from "what needs to change" to "what that change will look like" (Durrant, 1993). This vision of change could be thought of as people's preferred directions in life (i.e., Where would you like to be headed in your life?). This line of questioning establishes a positive momentum, makes workers' efforts more relevant to people's lives, and builds stronger helping relationships.

The second typical question "What caused this problem?" is firmly embedded in a belief that knowing what caused a problem will help us figure out how to best address it. This may or may not be the case. There are a number of possible descriptions of why someone has a problem and our hypotheses about possible causes may have little to do with effectively addressing the problem. In fact, most of the "answers" we have traditionally come up with have focused on deficits and are often experienced by people and families as blaming and shaming. It's a bit like starting our helping work by first digging a very deep hole, jumping into it with the people we intend to help, and then trying to form a relationship as we climb out. Could there be a better way? Thinking in terms of constraints may offer an alternative. When applied to problems in life, this idea shifts the organizing question from "What caused the problem?" to "What constrains a person or family from living differently?" Other ways of asking this question would be "What gets in the way of you doing things differently?" or "What pulls you away from how you'd prefer to be?" or "What obstacles or challenges stand in the way of the life you'd rather have?" We will generally refer to constraints as obstacles. Obstacles are those things that get in the way of the people living out the lives they'd prefer.

This combination flips our usual organizing questions from "What is the problem and what caused it?" to "Where would you like to be headed in your life and what gets in the way of that?" But we can go even further. Solution-focused approaches have suggested that we can help people without focusing on problems by devoting attention to those things that support them moving forward in their lives (deShazer, 1985). In our own experience, sometimes we can work with people to develop a vision and move directly into what supports them in moving forward. Other times that is not enough. Then we need to examine obstacles that stand in the way and help people directly deal with those challenges. With this in mind, we introduce four questions that make up the Collaborative Helping map in its simplest form:

> Where would you like to be headed in your life?
> What helps you get there?
> What gets in the way?
> What needs to happen next?

The Collaborative Helping map is illustrated in Figure 3.1.

Of course, helping work is infinitely more complex than simply asking people these four questions, receiving their thoughtful responses, and then watching them head off to live happily ever after. These four questions represent areas to be jointly explored. As highlighted in the last chapter, this is a process of collaborative inquiry where workers ask people questions to help them explore these four areas. The art and skill of this work lies in the ability to ask questions that are close to people's experience, are personally meaningful to them, and also stretch them beyond their automatic responses to go further in their own thinking and feeling. The next sections examine each of these areas in detail, providing guidelines for exploration and illustrating them with an example of a family involved with a home-based outreach team.

FIGURE 3.1   **OVERVIEW OF COLLABORATIVE HELPING MAP**

Vision	
Where would you like to be headed in your life?	
Obstacles/Challenges	**Supports**
What gets in the way?	*What helps you get there?*
Plan	
What needs to happen next?	

THE COLLABORATIVE HELPING MAP IN ACTION

Consider the following situation. Camila is a 14-year-old Latina girl with an infectious laugh, an outgoing personality, and talents in dance and drawing. She is also struggling with impulsivity and depression, and is escalating out of control behavior. She lives on the edge with a lot of risky behaviors that involve sex, drugs, and late-night partying with a crowd that scares her mother Rachel. Rachel is originally from Costa Rica and had Camila at age 14 shortly after coming to the United States. Rachel's parents have both passed away, but she remains close to her younger sister, Silvia, who lives nearby. Camila's father is out of the picture, as are the different fathers of her three younger siblings. The family lives in a poor urban neighborhood and is involved with a home-based, outreach team, Child Protective Services (due to previous charges of neglect), and Juvenile Probation (due to Camila's vandalism charges). Camila and Rachel have an explosive relationship. Rachel is worried that Camila is going to end up pregnant, in jail, or dead on the street. She fears that she will have to watch her daughter go through struggles she endured in coming to the United States. She often phones workers in crisis and has a tendency to exaggerate the stories she tells about Camila in the hopes that someone will grasp the severity of the situation. Camila is very reactive to her mother's exaggerations and minimizes concerns about her life decisions. The crowd she hangs out with has little use for adults, and Camila experiences a lot of pressure to be cool and suspicious of adults. She struggles to find a balance between peer expectations and her own cultural upbringing of close connection among different generations.

John, a Spanish-speaking Anglo worker, went out to meet with the family. He explained that he would like to use the first meeting to get to know them outside their immediate concerns. He asked about family traditions, how they spent time together, and what they were proud of about themselves as a family. He spent time with Rachel, listening to her worries and complaints about her daughter, and went for a walk with Camila, listening to her outrage at her mother's exaggerations about her behavior and hearing about her desire for more trust. This initial work was crucial to the success of their subsequent work. Relational connection is the heart of this work and needs to be attended to always. John's initial effort to get to know the family outside their immediate concerns built connection and ultimately saved time. It also provided an easy transition from stories of pride into hopes for a preferred direction in life. From those hopes, John was able to identify obstacles and supports and develop a plan with Rachel and Camila to draw on supports to address obstacles to help them realize the vision they had developed. The map they completed over several meetings is illustrated here, and each component is discussed in some detail.

ORGANIZING VISION AND PREFERRED DIRECTIONS IN LIFE

Our work with individuals and families often goes better when it is organized around preferred directions in life. A focus on possibilities (what life *could* look like rather than what is *wrong*) can lift people out of the immediacy of problems and provide a better foundation for responding to challenges. Clear vision can become an irresistible magnet that provides inspiration and direction. Eliciting a vision of possibilities implicitly conveys that alternatives are possible and, when traced out in detail, provides clues about the path to get there. Developing a vision together is also a way to collaboratively develop goals. As helpers we often hold models in our head about how people and families should function, which are inevitably influenced by our own values. But if we begin with people developing a vision of their own desired lives, that vision can guide our helping efforts from the start. In this way, the development of envisioned possibilities enhances collaboration and keeps our work focused and accountable to the people we serve.

The development of a proactive vision can be a process of eliciting hopes for the future (e.g., "What kind of person do you hope your daughter will be when she grows up? What makes those dreams for her particularly important to you? What do you think you need to do in your own life to help those hopes come true?"). This way of talking with people can also be used to focus on preferred ways of coping in a difficult present (e.g., "As your daughter continues to struggle with impulsivity, how would you like to respond to her? What would be important to you about responding in that way? What could help you respond in that way regardless of any surprises this situation might throw at all of you?"). In this way, the development of a proactive vision acknowledges problems in life and focuses on preferred ways of being in the face of difficulties. A focus on possibilities does not ignore problems but comes at them from outside their immediacy. This actually saves time and makes for more effective work. As Andrew Turnell (2008) has said, "It's a long day on the golf course if you don't know where the hole is."

As we ask people about preferred directions in life, it is important to keep in mind that we may be asking people stuck in a problem-filled life to imagine things that could seem out of their realm of possibilities. To make matters worse, the general expectation in seeking or being assigned help is that the focus will be on problems. This alternative way of approaching obstacles may be a bit of a stretch at first. As a result, it is important to provide a clear explanation of why we are starting in this fashion and to take difficulties in stride as we begin to establish a collaborative helping relationship.

Let's see how this went with Rachel and Camila. In his second meeting with them, John asked them about shared hopes for their life together. The conversation initially slid into an escalating confrontation about their respective complaints, but John stayed focused on their hopes for what could be different and eventually pieced together a mutual desire for a better relationship, more positive interactions, and shared trust and respect in which Camila wanted her mother to "be less on her back and trusting her more;" and Rachel wanted her daughter to "learn from Rachel's own mistakes and respect and listen to her more." Figure 3.2 shows the organizing vision they developed together (quotation marks highlight their words) along with some guidelines that can organize the development of such visions.

FIGURE 3.2   **ORGANIZING VISION IN THE COLLABORATIVE HELPING MAP**

Organizing Vision
Where would you like to be headed in your life?
Developing a mutually shared, proactive, meaningful, and sufficiently concrete vision Built on a foundation of motivation, resourcefulness, and community
We want to "get more trust and respect in our family." We both realize that Trust and Respect "are tied up together and that we both have to work to make this happen." In particular, Camila will work to "act more respectfully" toward Rachel and Rachel will work to "hold more trust in her daughter."
This is important because we miss the closeness we used to have when it was "us against the world." We can't think of many times right now where there has been more Trust and Respect but believe we have had some and are committed to building more. Other people who would notice and support this include Aunt Silvia (who is kind of an interpreter between us) and Camila's dance teacher, who Rachel trusts and Camila respects.

Important Components of an Organizing Vision

This organizing vision has a number of important qualities. It is mutually shared, proactive, meaningful, and sufficiently concrete. Let's briefly consider each of these in turn. While Camila and Rachel began with very different changes that they thought the other should make, John was able to keep them focused on their shared hopes and weave them together in a way that was acceptable to both. One of the biggest barriers to effective helping work is the lack of a shared focus. Things go better when everyone is pulling in the same direction and it is important to take the time initially to develop a focus that will help accomplish just that.

This vision is also proactive or forward thinking. It highlights particular activities that Camila and Rachel will begin doing. It is much easier to pursue a goal of something you are going to start doing rather than something you are going to stop doing. For example, consider the difference between a resolution to stop drinking after work and the resolution to start exercising instead of drinking after work. A decision to not do something leaves us in a void and often leaves us thinking about the activity we're trying to avoid. A goal of ending an undesirable behavior keeps us locked in the problem. A goal of beginning a new behavior invites people to step outside the problem's influence, opens new possibilities, and provides direction. When people initially frame goals or visions in terms of stopping or not doing something, we can ask them to flip that to tell us about what might be happening instead. This leads to proactive, forward-thinking goals.

The organizing vision developed by Camila and Rachel is meaningful and concrete. They talked with sadness about the closeness they used to have. The words "trust" and "respect" resonated with a deep relational connection between them despite their fiery blowups. Chip and Dan Heath (2007) have drawn from a creative mix of marketing, psychology, urban legends, and Aesop's fables to coin the phrase "sticky messages." By this they mean simple, unexpected, concrete, credible, emotional stories that capture and hold people's attention. We can apply the notion of sticky messages to the process of helping people develop a shared vision that captures their imagination and attention. As one mother involved with CPS put it, "My worker initially spent time with me asking about my hopes for my kids in a way that brought tears to my eyes. We developed a simple bumper sticker 'better together whatever' that sounds kind of dumb, but held incredible meaning for me. She then framed our ongoing service planning in terms of that phrase and it all made so much more sense to me. I was totally on board and we got a lot more work done together." People who have a clear vision for the future cope better with challenging current situations. If we think about an organizing vision as a lighthouse serving as a beacon in dark times, it is crucial that the vision be bright enough to be seen through the fog of everyday life and close enough to people's everyday experience to be noticeable. It is also helpful if the vision captures people's imaginations to serve as an inspiration for future action. Here are some examples of bumper sticker visions that have come to hold significant meaning for the people developing them:

- I want to be the boss of my feelings rather than have my feelings be the boss of me (from an 11-year-old angry girl)
- Do the right thing rather than do things right (from a man trapped in a bureaucratic job)
- Love, not lies (from a couple with a long history of deceit about substance use)

It is important to help people develop a clear vision that is as concrete as possible. To the extent that a vision of preferred directions in life serves as a beacon of hope, it will be more effective if it is concrete and specific. When we are helping people develop a vision to guide shared work, it is important to ask detailed questions that flesh out the vision. Some questions to help do that might include:

- Concretely, what would that look like?
- Can you say more about that aspect you've just described?
- If we had a video of this future you're describing, what would we see on it?
- If I were a fly on the wall noticing this, what would I see?

It is important to pursue this line of questioning with genuine curiosity and get a detailed story of this possible future.

Solution-focused approaches have emphasized the importance of helping people develop goals that are achievable (Berg, 1994; Berg & Miller, 1992). A focus on future possibilities invites hope and a sense of movement. Goals that are too large or difficult to achieve can quickly sabotage that movement. At the same time, helping professionals often sell people short and encourage people to be "realistic." We might say, "Your son wants to be a rock star but can't get out of bed in the morning. Let's get real here" or "Your daughter has been diagnosed with a thought disorder and probably will never hold down a job in her life. You have to accept that." We think it is important to dream big and then use that dream as a starting point to narrow our focus in the interest of getting real. Here is an example of setting realistic goals.

> Alex was a 14-year-old White youth diagnosed with Asperger's syndrome. He had trouble reading social cues and was often wildly inappropriate in his interactions with others. He had a dream of becoming a sports agent representing NBA basketball players. His parents were supportive of this, despite input from numerous psychiatrists who cautioned them that Alex's condition would make it difficult for him to find any job, let alone a public relations job. An outreach worker who had been instructed by her supervisor to help Alex and his parents develop a more realistic appraisal of the situation took an approach instead of "dream big, get real" to elicit Alex's initial vision of representing Kobe Bryant (a well-known Los Angeles basketball star) and traced out the hopes and dreams behind that vision. She then examined with Alex possibilities that could make that dream come true as well as real-life challenges that could complicate that dream. In the process, Alex highlighted the importance of statistics in promoting stars and showed his intimate knowledge of sports statistics acquired through the Internet. A conversation about his love of Internet statistics and his dread of interpersonal encounters led to a developing appreciation that perhaps his contribution to sports superstar representation might be best fostered through an accumulation of background statistics rather than foreground representation. He shifted his career aspirations from representing sports superstars (in his words, "being a showboat") to supporting the representation of sports superstars (in his words, "helping the showboats look knowledgeable").

In this instance, the emergent vision with Alex and his family began big and became realistic.

Finally, we can strengthen the hold of an organizing vision by asking questions that build a foundation of *motivation* (Why is this vision important to you?), *resourcefulness* (When have you been able to bring bits of this vision into your life?), and *community* (Who in your life or work appreciates this vision and has supported you or might support you in the future in grounding your life here more often?). These three areas help to solidify the vision. The second half of the vision developed by Rachel and Camila captures their responses to these questions and helps solidify their vision and give it more substance in their shared life.

OBSTACLES AND SUPPORTS

Once we have a clear vision and a foundation of motivation, resourcefulness, and community, we can ask people about some of the challenges or obstacles they may encounter on the road to a preferred future as well as what might support or contribute to them getting there. We can be flexible and ask people if they would prefer to start with obstacles or supports. This allows us to move in the direction of what is most important to them.

Some examples of obstacles could include behavioral health problems (e.g., depression, hyperactivity, tantrums); common feelings (e.g., sadness, anger, frustration); beliefs (e.g., my son is bad, I am worthless, there is no hope for us); interactional patterns between family members (e.g., the more a father corrects his son, the more the son rebels and the more the son rebels, the more his father corrects him); real-life dilemmas (e.g., If I confront my husband about his infidelity, he will leave me penniless. If I don't, I will hate myself); unavoidable situations (e.g., generational poverty or lack of education); and broader cultural forces (e.g., racism, sexism, classism, heterosexism).

While the helping field has typically focused more on problems and obstacles, we can also help people identify supports. These may include sustaining habits and practices (e.g., meditating, exercising, or counting to five before responding to one's children); sustaining beliefs (e.g., I can make a difference in my life); sustaining interactional patterns among family members (e.g., a father's validation and acknowledgment of his son leads to the son being more open and forthcoming and vice versa); intentions, purposes, values, hopes, and dreams (e.g., love for one's children, a desire to be a better parent, a commitment to sobriety); supportive community members; and broader sustaining cultural expectations (e.g., a cultural value for respect and family).

The Collaborative Helping map encourages identification of obstacles and supports at individual, relational, and sociocultural levels (sociocultural level here refers to both a community level and broader social, cultural, economic, and political levels). It is useful to talk with people about obstacles in ways that help to *separate* the problem from the person and to talk about supports in ways that help to *connect* the person to their better intentions and sense of agency. Let's explore what this means.

In talking about obstacles and problems, it is important to do this in ways that minimize blame and shame. Blame and shame shut down conversations and limit possibilities because they trigger defensiveness. As a result, it becomes crucial to find ways of talking about problems that don't meld them with people's identities. If we can find ways to talk about problems that leaves some space for people to experience themselves outside the influence of shame and blame, we will save considerable time and energy. In an era of reduced funding and cost containment, who can argue with finding ways to make our work more efficient and effective?

Usefulness of Externalizing Problems

One way to do this kind of helping talk draws on the practice of externalizing from narrative approaches. Externalizing conversations were originally developed by Michael White and David Epston (1990) as a way to talk with people about problems as separate from them in order to help them hold on to a sense of self outside the influence of those problems. Historically, our field has thought about people as *having* a problem (e.g., I suffer from depression) or *being* a problem (e.g., I'm a depressed person). In both instances, the problem is internalized and mixed up with people's identity. Externalizing is a way of thinking about problems that views people as being in a *relationship with* a problem (e.g., Depression has come into my life and has made a mess of it for me) rather than having or being a problem. This relationship is a *two-way relationship*. The problem has influence in the life of the person and important others around him/her and the person has influence in the life of the problem.[1] This relationship is *ongoing*. There is a history and context to it. We can examine times when the problem has more influence in the life of the person and what supports that as well as times when the person has more influence in the life of the problem and what supports that. Finally, this relationship is *changeable*. There is always life outside of the problem (even though that may be very hard to see at times) and no problem has total control over a person's life.

This alternative way of thinking about problems holds a number of distinct advantages for the helping process. The separation of people and problems can alleviate the immobilizing effects of shame and blame and reduce defensiveness. When people experience themselves as being in a relationship with a problem rather than having or being a problem, they often experience a sense of relief and an increased ability to do something about the problem. In this way, externalizing creates a space between people and problems, which enables them to draw on previously obscured abilities, skills, and know-how to revise their relationship with the problem. Externalizing also provides a way to untangle the tight knot of blame and responsibility. While our field (and popular culture) has historically sought to get people to "own the problem" and take responsibility for it, externalizing creates a separation that, in a sense, blames the problem for its effects while helping people take responsibility for their responses to those effects. Karl Tomm (1989) has framed this issue in the following way.

> Externalizing doesn't remove personal responsibility. It focuses and refines it. People are invited to recognize that they have the option of continuing to submit to the influence of externalized problems or the option of rejecting the invitation to submit to the dictates of the problem. As they begin to see these alternatives more clearly and experience them as genuine options, they almost invariably select the latter. They are, of course, then supported in their protest and rebellion against the oppression of the problem.

Externalizing can also help workers develop a more compassionate view of people who engage in off-putting behaviors. For example, when we think of a particular person as being captured by emotions such as rage or hurt or frustration rather than as being rageful or histrionic or frustrating, we may have a more empathic response to them. We can see the way in which the Rage, the Hurt, or the Frustration gets hold of them and disrupts their life, our working relationship, and our own experience of being with them.[2] From this perspective, we can perhaps view this as an unfortunate situation we are in together rather than feeling animosity toward them or feeling ineffective in our work as a helper. This can be particularly useful in situations in which both parties are overextended and undersupported. Again, as we just highlighted, blaming the problem does not exonerate the person from holding responsibility for how they respond to the ways in which a particular problem might invite or encourage them to behave.

Finally, externalizing assumptions can offer a way to move beyond being either problem focused or solution focused. Strength-based approaches are often subjected to the criticism that they romanticize families and minimize any discussion of real problems. The process of externalizing provides a way of thinking that both acknowledges problems (while viewing people as distinct from them) and focuses our attention on people's ability to develop a different relationship with those problems. Externalizing provides a way to acknowledge people's experience of problems without inadvertently contributing to blame and shame.

Identifying Obstacles with Collaborative Helping Maps

Again, let's return to Rachel and Camila and see how John helped them to identify obstacles to and supports for the vision they had developed together. John asked them what could pull them away from their shared desire for Trust and Respect. Rachel identified Camila's impulsiveness and Camila identified Rachel's constant worrying. John subtly changed their descriptions from adjectives to nouns and asked how the Impulsivity and the Worry could be obstacles to their vision of "Trust and Respect." He also asked about the effects of those problems on Camila, Rachel, and their relationship. As they responded, John wondered whether Impulsivity and Worry might be connected in some way. Camila and Rachel described intense arguments in which Rachel's expressions of concern grew into "accusations and bringing up the past" and invited Camila's "denial and threats to hurt herself to get her mother to back off," which led to more concern on Rachel's part and on and on. They disagreed about the cause of these fights ("I explode because my mom nags me and drives me crazy." "No, I nag because my daughter explodes and doesn't take me seriously."). However, they both agreed that the fights were stressful and left them each feeling "disrespected and raw." John asked whether the interaction might be like a dance that could take on a life of its own and they both agreed with that description. They worked out a title for the dance as that "Nag/Explode Thing." Rachel and Camila were clear they did not like that "Nag/Explode Thing" and thought it did great damage to their relationship. Finally, John attempted to place Impulsivity, Worry, and that Nag/Explode Thing in a broader sociocultural context and asked whether Camila and Rachel knew other mothers and daughters who had similar struggles and what other pressures mothers and daughter might be under as they try to negotiate the interface of cultures. Camila talked about her "American" friends giving her grief for being so close to her mother and encouraging her to "grow up and lie" so that she could go out with them. John wondered whether Camila's friends might be channeling this American adolescent idea that "Kids are cool and parents drool," which brought a smile and appreciative nod from Camila. Rachel talked about some of her friends being aghast that she "allowed" her daughter to talk back to her. John wondered whether that might be tied to a strong cultural idea that parents "should be in control of their kids." Rachel responded that she felt like she "should" be in control of Rachel and that she also knew Camila had a stubborn streak (which she admired) and wasn't likely to be controlled by anyone. Figure 3.3 outlines the obstacles and supports section of their Collaborative Helping map.

FIGURE 3.3   **OBSTACLES AND SUPPORTS IN THE COLLABORATIVE HELPING MAP**

Obstacles *What gets in the way of Trust and Respect?*	**Supports** *What supports Trust and Respect?*
Identifying obstacles at individual, relational, and sociocultural levels Described in a way that *separates* problems from people	Identifying supports at individual, relational, and sociocultural levels Described in a way that *connects* people to their better intentions and sense of agency
Impulsivity that gets Camila in trouble at school and with her mom. **Worries** that make it hard for Rachel to trust her daughter. That **Nag/Explode Thing**—Rachel's expressions of Worries lead to Camila's Explosions and exacerbate Worries. Possible **adolescent cultural belief** in which friends encourage "**separation**" and "dissing" of adult culture. Possible **parent cultural belief** that parents should have **control** over their children and attempt to exert that control in problematic ways.	Camila's **openness** to getting help. Rachel's **commitment** to her daughter and **welcoming of supports**. **Connection** between Camila and Rachel and their desire to recapture the **closeness** they used to have. **Aunt Silvia** as someone who provides a place for Camila to stay when things heat up between Rachel and Camila and as an interpreter who is trusted by both parties. **Dance and art** as activities after school that engage Camila and help her keep busy and out of trouble.

In this way, John elicited externalized obstacles at an individual level (Impulsivity and Worry), at a relational level (that Nag/Explode Thing), and at a broader sociocultural level (a cultural "should" about adolescent separation that can divide teens and their parents and a cultural "should" about parental control that can encourage problematic interactions between parents and youth). He examined the effects of these externalized problems on Camila, Rachel, and their relationship, and ways in which these problems were obstacles to their desire for "Trust and Respect."

Identifying Supports with Collaborative Helping Maps

John also asked Rachel and Camila about things that supported Trust and Respect in their life together. At an individual level, they identified Camila's openness to getting help and Rachel's commitment to her daughter and welcoming of support from others. At a relational level, they identified Aunt Silvia as an interpreter who understood Camila and respected Rachel. They thought she could provide a place for Camila to "run to" that Rachel could tolerate. They also identified dance and drawing as after-school activities that engaged Camila and helped her keep busy and out of trouble.

It is useful to identify supports in ways that highlight intentionality and help to foster a sense of agency (an experience that one is initiating and executing one's own volitional actions in the world or, to use a story metaphor, that one has more influence and participation as the author of one's own life story). This requires a shift in how we think about "strengths." We can move from thinking about strengths as essential qualities that reside inside of people (characteristics or "who" people are) to considering them as skills of living (practices or "how" people are) that are guided by people's intentions, values and beliefs, hopes and dreams, and commitments in life. This shift can lead to richer conversations and enhance people's sense of personal and collective agency. We examine it in more depth in Chapter 6.

For now, let's focus on Camila's previously described openness to help. We could think about this "openness to help" as a characteristic (i.e., she's an open person). We could also think about this "openness to help" as a practice in living (e.g., How does Camila "do" openness? What are the practices of this openness? How did she develop these practices? Who and what supported her in that process?). As John invited Camila to trace out the ways in which she actively sought out help, he elicited a story of the specific ways in which she did that. This allowed John to ask Camila what her intentions were in seeking out help ("I don't like what my life looks like and I want something different."). That response allowed John to ask Camila about the values and beliefs that stood behind that intention ("People should have a say in their lives and be able to draw on those who care about them."). That response allowed John to ask Camila about the hopes and dreams that stood behind those values ("I want a life where I'm making choices and those choices are respected and acknowledged by others."). While this shortened version can present Camila as an extremely insightful person (which she was), it's important to not underestimate the contribution of John's patient and disciplined, yet conversational, questioning in this process. The questions we ask shape the responses we get and this particular questioning process can evoke a very powerful experience in a very short time. It brings us back to the idea from Chapter 2 about definitional ceremonies. As helpers, our interactions with people have the potential to open possibilities for different experiences of self to emerge, leading to different life stories that are told and lived out by them. In this way, John opened space for Rachel and Camila to experience themselves and their relationship quite differently. They were describing strengths and supports in a much richer way, but more important, they were experiencing their lives in a way that opened more possibilities for them.

THE PLAN

The final part of the Collaborative Helping map brings responses to the first three questions together into a practical and holistic query, "What needs to happen?" The goal of this section is to develop a meaningful, proactive, mutually agreed-upon plan that draws on supports to address obstacles to achieve the vision and outlines concrete steps that each participant will take. You'll notice the parallel in the vision and plan sections of developing something that is mutually shared, proactive, meaningful, and concrete. The rationales highlighted for these qualities in the vision section also hold for the plan section. It is important to engage people's natural communities in developing and supporting collaboratively developed plans. If we truly understand that people live in social networks and appreciate the potential of community, we must actively recruit important family and friends who are all around the people we are helping.

FIGURE 3.4   **PLAN IN THE COLLABORATIVE HELPING MAP**

> **Plan**
> *Who will do what, when, and with whom*
> *to draw on supports and address obstacles to "live into" vision?*
>
> Developing a meaningful, proactive, mutually agreed-upon plan that draws on supports to address obstacles to achieve vision.
> Outlining an action plan that concretely specifies who will do what.
> Engaging people's natural community to support a plan.
>
> In order to support the development of Trust and Respect in our family:
> - Camila will talk with John to examine the impact of Impulsivity on her life and what she wants to do about that. Rachel will talk with John to examine the impact of Worry on her life and find ways to turn down its volume without completely turning it off.
> - Rachel and Camila will develop a plan for Camila to go to Aunt Silvia's when necessary to provide a space that interrupts that Nag/Explode Thing.
> - Camila and Rachel will talk with John about ways to untie the knot of Impulsivity and Worry.
> - John will help Camila find dance and art classes after school to keep her engaged, occupied, and out of trouble to support the development of Trust and Respect. He will also help to arrange for transportation and find funding for these classes through an agency flexible fund.
> - John will help Rachel reconnect to a knitting group she used to belong to and will provide transportation for her to that group for the first 2 months.
> - Camila and Rachel will talk with John to examine some of the broader sociocultural supports for Impulsivity, Worry, and that Nag/Explode Thing and figure out what they want to do about that.

This goes far beyond typical requirements for routine service planning. The plan section for Rachel and Camila is highlighted in Figure 3.4.

As you look at the different components of this plan, you'll notice that it seeks to pull in some of the broader community around Camila and Rachel (e.g., Aunt Silvia and Rachel's knitting group) and that it includes both concrete services and things to be talked about. The incorporation of a broader network moves helping efforts from simply providing services to drawing on people's existing communities of support. Network therapists draw a distinction between primary networks—the extended family, friends, and important others in someone's life—and secondary networks—the professional network that is paid to be in someone's life (Kliman & Trimble, 1983). We like this distinction because it reminds us of our place as paid helpers. We are secondary and our role is to identify, gather, and support people's primary networks in helping them.

The integration of concrete services with meaningful conversations fits with our previously discussed metaphor of "walking and talking." As an outreach worker, John has the luxury of being available for more than just a 50-minute hour once a week, and this significantly contributes to his helpfulness with families. Many of his best conversations have occurred when engaging in concrete activities or driving people around. He helped Camila find and enroll in after-school classes, initially took her there, then helped her arrange for transportation there and back, and found ways to pay for the classes through a flexible funding account, which is an important feature of many outreach programs. The time immediately after school was the time Rachel was most likely to get into trouble and the payment for after-school classes to keep her out of trouble at that time is a very good investment for funding sources. Rachel had expressed a desire to return to an old knitting group that she had dropped out of in order to be at home when Camila returned from school. Camila's participation in after-school classes opened up the possibility for Rachel to return to the knitting group and get informal peer support from other mothers (probably more normalizing and useful for her than the formal support of a parenting group for mothers with problems). She was nervous about going, and John agreed to go with her and drive her there until she became more comfortable (although he was initially teased mercilessly by the other women in the group). These concrete helping efforts made him much more relevant to Camila and Rachel's lives and also afforded many opportunities for thoughtful, though informal, conversations with a goal of helping them experience themselves differently and live out their preferred life stories. We examine the process of doing this in more detail in Chapter 6. For now let's take a look at the entire map and reflect on its usefulness as shown in Figure 3.5.

This map, developed over the first few meetings, became a road map for John's work with Camila and Rachel. It provided a touchstone for all of them to come back and see whether their work together was on track and headed in an agreed-upon direction. It's important to keep in mind that these maps are a dynamic work in progress rather than a static product. In the course of revisiting them, they often change as the conditions of life change. They provide an organizing focus for our work and are most useful as a flexible working document.

FIGURE 3.5   COMPLETED COLLABORATIVE HELPING MAP

Organizing Vision
Where would you like to be headed in your life?

We want to "get more trust and respect in our family." We both realize that Trust and Respect "are tied up together and that we both have to work to make this happen." In particular, Camila will work to "act more respectfully" toward Rachel and Rachel will work to "hold more trust in her daughter."

This is important because we miss the closeness we used to have when it was "us against the world." We can't think of many times right now where there has been more Trust and Respect but believe we have had some and are committed to building more. Other people who would notice and support this include Aunt Silvia (who is kind of an interpreter between us) and Camila's dance teacher, who Rachel trusts and Camila respects.

Obstacles	Supports
What gets in the way of Trust and Respect?	*What supports Trust and Respect?*
Impulsivity that gets Camila in trouble at school and with her mom.	Camila's **openness** to getting help.
Worries that make it hard for Rachel to trust her daughter.	Rachel's **commitment** to her daughter and **welcoming of supports**.
That **Nag/Explode Thing**—Rachel's expressions of Worries lead to Camila's Explosions and exacerbate Worries.	**Connection** between Camila and Rachel and their desire to recapture the **closeness** they used to have.
Possible **adolescent cultural belief** in which friends encourage "**separation**" and "dissing" of adult culture.	**Aunt Silvia** as someone who provides a place for Camila to stay when things heat up between Rachel and Camila and as an interpreter who is trusted by both parties.
Possible **parent cultural belief** that parents should have **control** over their children and attempt to exert that control in problematic ways.	**Dance and art** as activities after school that engage Camila and help her keep busy and out of trouble.

Plan
Who will do what, when, and with whom to realize this vision?

In order to support the development of Trust and Respect in our family:
- Camila will talk with John about the impact of Impulsivity on her life and what she wants to do about that. Rachel will talk with John about the impact of Worry on her life and find ways to turn down its volume without completely turning it off.
- Rachel and Camila will develop a plan for Camila to go to Aunt Silvia's when necessary to provide a space that interrupts that Nag/Explode Thing.
- Camila and Rachel will talk with John about ways to untie the knot of Impulsivity and Worry.
- John will help Camila find dance and art classes after school to keep her engaged and occupied to support the development of Trust and Respect.
- John will help Rachel reconnect to a knitting group that was very important to her.
- Camila and Rachel will talk with John to examine some of the broader sociocultural supports for Impulsivity, Worry, and that Nag/Explode Thing and figure out what they want to do about that.

THE USEFULNESS OF A MAP

We have talked at length about a new way of organizing our thinking about helping efforts. Collaborative Helping maps grow out of a principled practice framework that takes people and helpers from vision through obstacles and supports until we arrive at a plan. The Collaborative Helping map can help keep both helpers and the people served oriented in shared work. While the map is not a magic pill that remedies the difficulties of the journey, it does give it direction and focus. It also provides a way for people on the journey to travel together with hope and a shared purpose. The use of these maps both helps workers develop habits of thought to work their way through complicated situations and a structure to guide conversations with people about challenging issues. Our experience with the use of these maps over time is that they result in helpers positioning themselves quite differently with people and taking up a spirit of respect, connection, curiosity, and hope. This chapter utilized an example from home-based outreach work. The next chapter examines applications of these maps in residential, child protective services, and home health care.

NOTES

1. We want to be clear here that we are not suggesting this is simply a mutual relationship and that there are not often significant power dynamics in the relationship between problems and people. Often problems in people's lives receive significant support from the broader context of our lives and it is important that we consider and address this larger context.
2. Throughout this book, when we are talking about a particular problem in an externalizing fashion, we will capitalize it.

CHAPTER 4

Collaborative Helping Maps in Different Contexts

While the previous chapter used an example of an outreach situation to introduce Collaborative Helping maps, these maps can also be used in many other contexts. This chapter highlights ways these maps can provide a conceptual guide for work across a wide variety of settings. In particular, it looks at how these maps have been used to focus assessment and treatment planning in a residential context and highlights ways helpers can promote constructive conversations with families involved with Child Protective Services. We also examine how Collaborative Helping maps may add value in health systems, which are paying increased attention to new methods of supporting people and families.

USING COLLABORATIVE HELPING MAPS IN RESIDENTIAL PROGRAMS

Residential treatment is filled with challenges and dilemmas for everyone involved. It becomes the depository of youth who can no longer live at home, having the paradoxical goal of simultaneously rescuing kids from problematic home situations and striving for the reunification of those same youth with the parents and/or caregivers who are often seen as the problem in the first place. Residential workers watch in utter frustration as children they have come to deeply care for sit on a front step waiting for a parent who does not arrive for a planned visit. Parents watch in anguish and anger as people hardly older than their children end up making decisions about their lives without a full understanding of the challenges of parenting in the real world. The combined situation, all too often, leads to evaluation, comparison, and competition over who might best contribute to the development of a particular child's life. Many innovative practitioners have attempted to counter this trend and build partnerships that support good outcomes for youth and families in difficult situations. Let's look at some ways in which Collaborative Helping maps might contribute to these efforts.

We'll begin with a story of work with a child and her family in an urban residential school. The program serves boys and girls from ages 6 to 14 and has youth for an average stay of around 8 months. Becca is a new social worker in the program who brings a lot of creativity and enthusiasm into her work. She carries an individual caseload and meets with children and their families as well as doing crisis management and larger system coordination with other involved workers.

She has been working with a two-parent Puerto Rican family that lives in a poor urban neighborhood. Eva is a 10-year-old girl who lives with her mother, Sylvia, stepfather, Enrique, and two siblings, Carlos (9) and Myrna (7). Enrique is steadily employed as a bus driver, while Sylvia has been intermittently employed in a variety of different jobs. They report that they get by, but it's often a challenge economically. Despite difficult times, the family is close and they care a great deal about each other. Eva is a large girl who is athletic and artistic. She was referred to the residential school due to a variety of mental health struggles. From a very young age, she had a history of wildly fluctuating mood swings with violent anger, often directed at her siblings who are physically much smaller than her. This was exacerbated by post-traumatic stress responses after witnessing a close friend killed by a stray bullet from a drive-by shooting on her school playground at age 6. Since that time, Eva has been in and out of residential and day programs with multiple hospitalizations.

At this point, the program was beginning to use Collaborative Helping maps as a routine part of their initial assessment and treatment planning. Becca describes some of her first contacts with Collaborative Helping maps.

> I'm pretty new to using Collaborative Helping maps. I haven't done them directly with families so much yet but use them to sort through my own thinking. The children and families we

work with have a lot going on and these maps are very useful to keep me organized and focused on what is my purpose and what am I doing here.

How is that useful to you in your work?

I think it's easy to go off on tangents in this work and be distracted by all the messiness of human lives and all the things we *could* talk about. And so, having a way to organize your thinking keeps it focused on a goal and you avoid getting caught up in distractions. For example, Eva's stepfather isn't her dad, but he is her siblings' dad. That could be a pretty compelling issue to explore, but is it relevant to the goal of her returning home? Maybe it is, but maybe not and if not, then we don't need to go into that. These maps keep us focused on what we've agreed to work on with the family and that builds a stronger relationship with them.

This residential program has found the Collaborative Helping map particularly helpful in organizing their assessment and treatment planning process with children and families.[1] We show the Collaborative Helping map that Becca completed with this family in Figure 4.1, highlight her comments about the usefulness of these maps for assessment and planning, and explore the broader usefulness of these maps in program functioning.

This was one of Becca's first maps. We wanted to use it to emphasize that these are works in progress rather than finished products. It was completed early on in Eva's stay in the program and reflects some of the early engagement challenges that faced the program with Eva's family. While Becca found the map very helpful to organize her thinking about engagement, assessment, and treatment planning, we can imagine how completing the map with the family as a joint initial assessment of their hopes for their life and Eva's stay at the program as well as their sense of obstacles to and supports for those hopes might enhance the engagement process.

Vision, Obstacles/Supports, Plan

Michael Durrant (1993), in a wonderful book on residential treatment, has reframed discharge from residential programs as readmission to life and highlighted the usefulness of viewing residential treatment as a

FIGURE 4.1   EVA'S COLLABORATIVE HELPING MAP

Organizing Vision
Where would you like to be headed in your life?
Eva and her family all want her to be able to return to live with them safely and permanently.

Obstacles	Supports
What gets in the way?	*What helps you get there?*
Eva's challenging behaviors and needs for extra support and structure	Commitment of Eva and her family to a common goal
Sylvia's own struggles with depression and anxiety and history with programs herself	Family love and support within both the nuclear and extended family
Financial pressures, child care needs, transportation difficulties	Ability to have positive visits together
	Stated parental openness to support services
Struggle to visit consistently, keep appointments, and remain available by phone to Eva and program staff	Eva's relational skills that sometimes allow her to work with trusted adults to help her get back on track and manage her difficult emotions, cope with stressors in her environment, get attention in positive ways, and stay on track
Lack of extended family support for Eva being in a residential program	
Pride that can get in the way of accepting services or asking for help	Eva's emerging ability to identify her feelings, come up with safe choices for herself (and for other children who might be struggling), and her developing sense of empathy for others
Feelings of hopelessness for the future	

Plan
What needs to happen next?

Eva's continued progress while at the program may help the family and Eva herself feel more hopeful about her ability to eventually return home, as well as also help Eva's parents feel more positive about what the program can offer.

Getting to know program staff better and seeing their daughter's progress may help Eva's parents feel more comfortable and be able to be more consistent with visits and meetings.

The support of the outreach team may be able to help mitigate some of the external barriers that get in the way of visits, meetings, and cell phone availability, including financial pressures, child care needs, and transportation difficulties.

Eva can use her goal of going home to help motivate her to practice new coping skills, talk about her feelings, and work to gain greater control of her behavior when she is upset.

Eva can be encouraged to build upon her relational strengths to help her manage her strong emotions more positively.

period of practice in which young people and their families have opportunities to experience themselves as competent and successful. This particular program has been very much organized around that proposition. Here are some of Becca's comments about how Collaborative Helping maps have supported those efforts.

> I think beginning with a vision or goal helps to develop a shared purpose and get people moving in the same direction. I like examining obstacles and supports in the context of an organizing vision. Honing in on obstacles that are immediately relevant to what we're doing and why we're involved with a family seems really helpful. It makes it clearer what we're talking about and why.
>
> The same is true for the supports section. Assessments often have a little section for strengths and you fill in stuff like "she likes art and plays basketball." All right, those are strengths, but how do they relate to the goals this family has for themselves. Placing strengths in the context of supports for an organizing vision makes our work relevant and insures all the pieces fit towards that goal.
>
> That's been helpful for our team, especially in terms of thinking about the strengths of a child or family that are directly useful and how to rally those strengths towards the goal. We can move from Eva is artistic to Eva can express herself through art when she can't do só verbally. And that has helped us become more creative in helping her use that as a tool to express anger without so many violent outbursts.

Information gathering in helping efforts across all contexts can often be a monumental undertaking. We collect huge amounts of information, most of it focused on problems and dysfunction. This process can be arduous for workers and demoralizing for families. Repeated questions about a litany of challenges can pull families into an experience of their life as filled with problems and either drag them down or provoke defensiveness. The process of framing problems as obstacles to a preferred direction in life helps information collection to become theme driven rather than an accumulation of every piece of available data about a family. This sequencing helps bring a laserlike focus to our work, avoids overly long assessments, and enhances partnerships with families by insuring that our work is experienced by them as more directly relevant to their lives.

This holds true for supports as well as obstacles. At times, strengths-based work can develop a reputation of talking about the "positives" in a superficial fashion. Recasting strengths in a context of supports for preferred directions in life makes discussions about them more immediately relevant and shifts those conversations from "nice talk" (Isn't Eva resourceful?) to "pragmatic talk" (What of that resourcefulness might help Eva and her family move toward their hopes for their life together?), which in turn can lead to concrete action.

Finally, the plan section of this initial map highlights the ways in which the development of these maps is better seen as an ongoing process rather than a one-time product. Its initial elements are focused on building a stronger relationship between the program and the family in order to build a foundation for future work together. It also highlights some of the specific steps that the program seeks to take to support the development of a stronger working relationship.

Working with Obstacles and Supports

Becca found that thinking about problems as separate from people enhanced the program's work with Eva and her family. While a number of obstacles were identified, Becca focused in on "Anger" in particular in her work with Eva and talked about how helping Eva to think about Angry Feelings as separate from herself was helpful.

> Externalizing has been particularly useful with kids like Eva who have really angry feelings. To them it feels like that's not them—that they are out of control and something has taken over. When you help kids develop the language to say, "Like okay Anger just got inside of you right now and is getting in the way. When Anger takes over and is driving the car, what do you look like? Do you like that? No? So, how can we help you make Anger sit in the backseat or still be there, but not be in charge anymore?"

And how has that affected her?

> It eases self-blame. She still has a lot of that because it's a tough habit to break, but I think it gives her more control because she's clear that she's trying to move from being bossed around by Anger to bossing around Anger. And kids love to be in charge and feel that control because so often they're the ones getting

bossed around. Giving that power back to them can be really helpful, especially for kids who have heard very different messages their whole life. It makes it not about them. It's not you can't be angry. You can, but let's help you keep it from getting you in so much trouble. It allows Anger, but helps her keep it in its place.

Much of the work with Eva in the residential program was focused around creating some distance between her and Angry Feelings in order to open possibilities for her to respond differently. The shift from Eva thinking about herself as an angry, defective person to someone in a relationship with Angry Feelings that can come in and mess up her life is both a powerful journey and at times one that is a bit daunting given her history. We don't want to minimize that history or the complexity of her feelings about it, but we do want to recognize the various ways in which her experience of herself and the story she tells about that might trap her in a particular way of being. This is where viewing Eva's placement in the residential school as an opportunity for her and her parents to practice some different ways of being and relating to the problems that have come into their lives becomes very useful.

Becca also elicited supports for the vision of reunification by focusing on exceptions, asking questions like "Can you think of a time when you were able to remind yourself to walk away? How did you do that? Can you tell me about that time? What happened? Wow, how'd you do that? What else did you do?" She began by focusing on small moments and expanding on them with an intention of helping Eva experience herself as more and more able to manage and respond to Angry Feelings. These efforts fit with our notion of "walking and talking" in this work. The focus is not on helping Eva develop insight into why she gets angry but talking with her about concrete steps she is taking to respond to Angry Feelings and brainstorming with her to further build on those steps with a focus on helping her experience herself differently in the process and gain more confidence in her ability to live out a different life story.

Becca also described how the focus on obstacles and supports enhanced her work with Eva's mother, Sylvia. She talked about the Hopelessness in Sylvia's life and moving from thinking about Sylvia as a hopeless person to thinking about Hopelessness coming in on Sylvia and receiving a lot of support in the process from broader sociocultural factors.

She described the pervasive effect of mother blame on Sylvia's parenting and her sense that "I screwed up and my daughter is fated to a lousy life." An effect of that "sense of fate" was a complete lack of trust that things could change. Becca found it helpful to locate that sense of fate in a broader context of sociocultural marginalization and a powerful belief that "People struggle, things don't get better, and that's the best you can hope for in life." While Becca is continuing to work on ways to bring considerations of these larger sociocultural forces into conversations with families, she noted that placing the Hopelessness in Sylvia's life in a larger context helped her develop more empathy for Sylvia and strengthened their relationship.

Next Steps

Becca also had a number of thoughts about how Collaborative Helping maps could be better integrated into her program.

> I think where we need to grow as a program is communicating this to the direct care staff and helping us all be using it. So, one of the big issues for Eva is struggling when she doesn't know whether her mom is coming for a visit or not. And her mom struggles with being consistent in that with all the other pressures in her life. And when she doesn't show up, it breaks the hearts of direct care staff. We could focus on this as an opportunity for them to play an active role in supporting a different story emerging. We could focus more on direct care staff letting the mother know how great it is when she does show up and what a contribution it makes to Eva's life. And I think that is really important because the real work of this program occurs in the hallways in everyday life.

Many residential programs work to narrow the gap between "milieu" work and "clinical" work. At the same time, there remain strong pressures for milieu staff to focus on the daily management of behavior within the program while clinical staff do the more esoteric "therapy" work. "Walking and talking" as a metaphor for our work provides a way to bring clinical concerns into what Becca calls the "hallways of everyday life" within a residential program. This provides a way to rebalance this work in a way that breaks down these divisions; better legitimizes the concrete, daily work of residential programs; and better integrates it into program thinking and action to also expand it out beyond the program itself to children's homes, families, and communities.

Shaheer is the program director who has worked tirelessly to develop a program that is more welcoming and engaging of children's family and community. Here are some of his comments related to the usefulness of these maps in that effort.

> In my core, I believe kids should be living their lives out in their communities and I don't want to see them in a residential program if at all possible. And it's not about having everything buttoned up nice and neat in order to move on. Instead it's about getting clear about what are the things that are so unsafe or problematic that they can't live at home and how can we impact those things. We can talk about next steps and that sort of thing, but once kids are safe enough to live at home, our job as a residential program is done. And using these maps has been helpful in doing that.

How so?

> They force us to think in a systematic and clear way about what needs to be different for this kid to be home with this family. Because otherwise it can be so overwhelming to sift through all the stories and information that gets brought to us and before you know it, months have gone by. This is a way that sets accountability from the very beginning on agreements of what we're working towards. It keeps us on our toes to make sure we're focused on what needs to be done.
>
> If that needs to be adjusted or tweaked, then we do that. But at least we've set a course and we're working towards it and it's pretty measurable, not like "He needs to be stable." Okay, concretely what does that mean and look like? We're trying to work in a way that is different here. And there are all these factors in our work that pull us away from that. We're pulled towards focusing on problems and diagnoses, towards being experts about other people's lives, and towards working in ways that make things easier for workers than for families. We struggle with that and these maps help pull us back to where we want to be and keep us honest.

So, you've been using these maps for 6 months. As you continue using these maps, how do you think that might affect your program?

> On a real concrete level, I think it will decrease lengths of stay. I really do because it highlights the things that need to be different and the things we can draw on to make that happen. And, it's not coming from us; it's coming from a collaborative process that's happening with the family. We're developing a direction that is specific and concrete and developed with the family and we can together then track the progress towards that.

This is a bold claim and while we have not yet collected systematic evidence to evaluate it, it fits with our experience of how the work can become more efficient and effective when guided by a focused vision that actively involves and engages families. Shaheer's emphasis on more responsive helping efforts provides a transition to the next section examining how these maps can support more constructive conversations about challenging issues.

USING COLLABORATIVE HELPING MAPS TO ENHANCE CONVERSATIONS IN CHILD PROTECTIVE SERVICES

Engaging people who feel threatened with the dissolution of their family on the heels of reports of neglect or abuse is among one of the greatest challenges in human services. Workers in Child Protective Services (CPS) walk a fine line between compassionate engagement of caregivers and holding clear bottom lines around children's safety. On top of this challenge, CPS workers are often demeaned and treated with disrespect and condescension by the rest of the system. They are continually subjected to a dual evaluation of "doing too little too late" and "intervening too much too soon." As an upper level manager in CPS once told Bill, "As an agency, we are charged with the never explicit task of protecting the general public from the fact that horrible things can happen to children and so when the news of a tragedy breaks, the outrage against us for letting that seep into community consciousness is enormous. If a house caught fire, there is no way that the fire department would be excoriated to the same extent that we are for letting that happen." While we have encountered a number of institutional practices that confirm the worst stereotypes about this group of beleaguered workers, we remain continually amazed by the commitment, dedication, and perseverance of many CPS workers. This section highlights some ways in which one CPS worker has taken ideas from Collaborative

Helping and used them to help her engage families amid these many challenges.

Beth is an experienced CPS worker who holds a deep commitment to actively engaging a child's family and community and working in partnership with them to assure safety, permanency, and well-being. While she strongly believes there is a time and place for the careful use of statutory authority (what she calls "Getting Big"), her preference is to avoid that whenever possible because as she puts it, "I don't think long-term change is as likely when you're Getting Big. I think change is more likely to occur with respect and questions, and so I use Getting Big only as a tool of last resort and it doesn't happen very often (twice in the last 2 years)."

Beth has brought Collaborative Helping maps into her work in a number of different ways.

> Sometimes it's just to get through a plan for this week. What's the vision for the next 7 days, what's going to get in the way of that, what's going to support that, and what's the plan? Other times, I use it to develop a bigger overarching vision that guides our work together (What are your hopes for your kids? What kind of childhood do you want them to have? Where do you want to be headed as a family?) and then use the rest of the map to move towards a plan to get there.

She has found the maps to be helpful in organizing work that can be very messy. Here is a description of how she does that.

> For example, you get into a family and everyone is there and 16 different things are going on at once—yelling and screaming, crying and blaming, and secrets, and everybody's talking all at once. And in the midst of that, I pull out that map and it just helps me calm down. I see it as a tool that helps us get somewhere and gives us some direction. We need to know where we're headed and how to get there. I mean it's not the solution to every problem. It's not going to solve the crisis in the Middle East, but I think it organizes the mess a little bit. You know what I mean? It gives me direction and it organizes the family's voice. I guess I'm kind of into that; this is your family, your kids. What do you want and how can I collaborate with you to help you get that? You've told me this is what you want for your family and I'm here to help support that.

Beth has created a carbon form of the Collaborative Helping Map as shown in Figure 4.2 that she uses to organize her conversations with families.

She take notes at every meeting beginning with the particular focus for the day, highlighting obstacles and supports for that focus, and capturing next steps to move forward in the plan section. At the end of the meeting, she tears off the carbon copy and leaves it with the family to capture what they had talked about in the meeting. She types the map into her case notes and puts the hard copy in the file. If a map is needed as a safety plan, she has families sign at the bottom, along with her signature, and then both parties have a signed copy instantly. This is a great example of the ways in which these maps can be directly incorporated into the structures of our work.

The inclusion of vision holds great possibilities in CPS work. Eliciting caregivers' hopes for their children's future enhances engagement and sets a tone for a more collaborative relationship. It offers opportunities for parents to step out of the immediacy of a problem-filled, crisis-ridden life and builds on their own hopes and dreams for their children. When we have asked parents questions about their hopes and vision for their children, they typically relate some version of "I hope my children would say their upbringing was safe, stable, and happy" (Root & Madsen, 2013). This is a caregivers' version, in their own language, of the federal mandate to work toward safety, permanency, and well-being. Pursuing a goal that caregivers have articulated is a much more efficient and

FIGURE 4.2   **A CARBON VERSION OF THE COLLABORATIVE HELPING MAP**

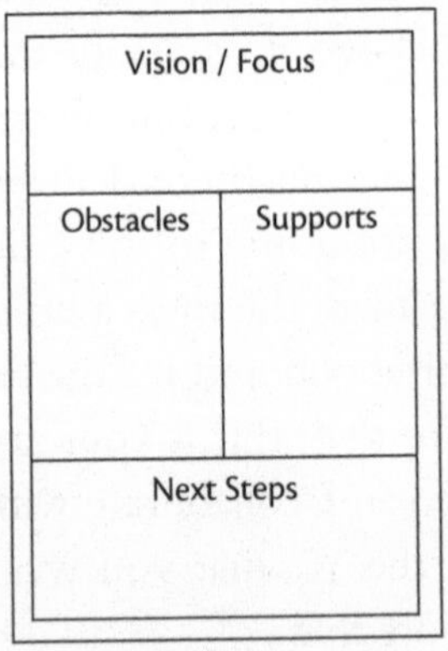

effective course of action. Vision is also a powerful intervention in its own right. As David Cooperrider (2000) has noted, "What we give attention to grows." Developing a strong vision and asking parents what makes that important to them, what small steps they have taken toward that vision, and who they can find to support them in further moving toward that vision, provides a foundation from which to honor their better intentions. Then, questions can more easily be raised about care-giver actions when they are inconsistent with those intentions.

Let's examine Beth's work with a White, working-class family. David is a 13-year-old boy who lives with his mother, Barb, stepfather, Art, and brothers, Sam (6) and Manny (2). The family became involved with CPS when it was reported that Art had hit David, resulting in bruises on his side and arms. Art had recently been released from prison for assault of someone outside the family and the local police became involved in the family interviews. David and his mother, Barb, were interviewed sepa-rately at school by Beth and a detective. Barb was cooperative and agreed to do what was needed to insure her children's safety. The detective and Beth then met with Art in jail. He was somewhat forthcoming and said he wanted to do what was "necessary to take care of the kids and do what was right." He described himself as "still being in prison mode when he didn't need to be" and agreed not to be alone with the kids until a thorough safety plan had been put in place upon his release.

Perhaps in all work with families, but particularly in CPS, it is crucial to keep an eye on the bottom line of safety, remembering why a child protection worker became involved in the first place and what it would take to "close the case." One way to keep issues that led to CPS involve-ment "on the table" is through the repeated use of scaling questions about danger and safety, asking everyone involved (family members and their broader network, CPS workers, and other involved helpers), "On a scale of 0 to 10 where 10 means everyone knows the children are safe enough for the child protection authorities to close the case and 0 means things are so bad that the children can't live at home, where do you rate this situation?" (Turnell, 2010). When different ratings are offered up, we can compare them and ask how various people make sense of these differences. We can also ask what is happening that allows them to give as high a rating as they did (which often highlights things that can fur-ther contribute to safety) and what it would take to move the rating up one number higher (which can help in safety planning).

Another way to support conversations about why we are involved in a family's life and what needs to happen next is through the use of harm and danger statements (Turnell & Parker, 2010). These written statements help social workers be explicit about their worries for a family. A harm statement is simply what was reported to authorities, framed in terms of caregiver actions and the resulting impact on the child. A danger statement is what the agency, social worker, and family are worried about happening in the future if changes are not implemented, again framed in terms of caregiver actions and impact on the child. Clear and concrete harm and danger statements help to maintain rapport during a difficult conversation, leading to more honest, respectful, and constructive discussions about what happened, why CPS is involved, and what they are worried about. Here are the statements Beth developed with the family.

Harm Statement: CPS received a report David had received bruises on his side and arms from being hit by Art. After the initial assessment, a second report was received stating that David had again been punched by Art and had bruises on his arm. During the course of the assessment, concern was also raised about Art's treatment of David, in particular that he was saying things that were hurtful and inappropriate.

Danger Statement: CPS, Barb, Art, and David are worried that without intervention, Art will continue to physically and emotionally abuse David, and he will suffer bruising and emotional harm.

More recently, Beth has been writing danger statements using externalizing language. Here is an example of one with this family.

Danger Statement: Beth, Barb, Art, and David are worried that without intervention, Prison Mode will again invade Art's better judgment, he will become angry and physically or emotionally abuse David, who will suffer bruising and emotional harm.

In this way, we are blaming Prison Mode rather than Art for the harm to his stepson, but also simultaneously holding Art accountable to change his relationship with Prison Mode in order to achieve the family goal of safely bringing the father back into the family. This shift to externalizing language allows Beth to partner with Art against Prison Mode in order to assure David's safety while working toward the family's goal of eventual reunification.

The use of harm and danger statements can lead directly into the formulation of safety goals—what we need to see in terms of changes in caregiver behavior and living arrangements to assure everyone that children are safe. These safety goals can then lead into specific safety plans developed by workers and family members to accomplish those goals. Here is Beth's description of how she puts all of this together.

> Harm and danger statements bring clarity to my work. They help me get clear about concrete, specific actions I am worried about and their impact on the child. They also help me have respectful and honest conversations with families about those worries. The danger statements lead pretty naturally into safety goals, which are just logical to have because that's why we're there and what we need to see to close the case. And then, I can use safety goals to go through a process of developing a concrete plan with a family for actions they will take to assure everyone that their children are safe.

We will look at the safety goals and safety plan that were actually developed with the family toward the end of this section. But first, let's examine how the use of Collaborative Helping maps with a particular focus on vision helped Beth get from these initial stages of clarifying harm and danger to engaging the parents in working toward safety goals. Beth has worked with families to develop vision statements, which are concise statements that capture and summarize their hopes and vision for their children and family that can then guide helping efforts while keeping a continual focus on safety.

Art's time in jail was difficult for the family. They were living on the edge of poverty with routine shut off notices and almost daily crises of one sort or another. Beth was providing a lot of concrete services to help out during this time (as well as referring them for therapy and other services). She was concerned about how Barb would be able to get through this time without falling into despair and how she could keep a focus on the children amid numerous crises. In that context, she worked with Barb to develop a vision statement. She asked a number of questions organized around this central query:

> Twenty years from now, what is the story you hope your children will tell about their childhood and your role in it?[2]

This was an extended conversation that required engaged curiosity, gentle persistence, and a foundation of relational connection. Here is the vision statement that emerged (framed in the children's words):

> Our life has been hard, but we've grown stronger because of it. Our mom did what she needed to do to protect us and to put a roof over our heads and food in our stomachs. She was nice and did what she needed to do to keep us safe and healthy. She did her best and stayed in contact with our teachers and was as involved as she could be in our activities. She told us that we could do anything we put our minds to.

Beth typed up this vision statement on a card, had it laminated, and gave it to Barb, who was very moved by it, read it to her children, and put it on her refrigerator. Here are some of Beth's hopes and intentions in undertaking this effort.

> I see it as a way to attend to the relationship between the family and me. I think that's an ongoing process that has to be given attention throughout the life of our work together. It's also a way of helping parents to step out of the immediacy of problems in their lives, connect to their better intentions and judgment, and give voice to what they want for their children. The thing that happened with David was significant and scary, especially given Art's previous conviction of felony assault and having recently gotten out of prison. Barb seemed determined to make her relationship with him work. At the same time, it was made very clear to her from both the cops and me that she needed to protect her children and she conveyed to me on a regular basis that she was willing to do whatever was needed to keep the kids safe. But when we work through "What it is you want for your kids and how do *you* want to be as a Mom?" we're giving her a voice and some control over a child protection worker being in her life. Often, CPS involvement is an adversarial process that can be very disempowering for parents and I have a commitment to doing it in a more collaborative way because I just think it is more effective.

One of Beth's adaptations of Collaborative Helping maps is what she calls "doing the vision." This is a process of pulling out the themes from a vision statement, writing them down on a piece of paper with space between them, and then over time going through each sentence and asking different family members how they see themselves putting that vision into practice.

The letter that follows (written shortly after Art was released from jail, living elsewhere, and only having supervised contact with his children) summarizes this work.

> Hi Barb and Art,
>
> Here is a summary of the conversation I had with Barb and the kids in August. I thought it was good conversation and wanted you to see it in writing.
>
> *Vision Statement:* "Our life has been hard, but we've grown stronger because of it. Our mom did what she needed to do to protect us and to put a roof over our heads and food in our stomachs. She was nice and did what she needed to do to keep us safe and healthy. She did her best and stayed in contact with our teachers and was as involved as she could be in our activities. She told us that we could do anything we put our minds to.
>
> 1. *How are you growing stronger?*
>   David said he is growing stronger by being a little less socially anxious. Barb said that Sam is being responsible for a few more chores. Barb said she is growing stronger by applying for a new job at the hospital. The family is stronger when school is out for the summer as everyone is helpful around the house. The family is continuing to share/voice their feelings and thoughts to each other.
> 2. *What is Mom doing to protect you, keep you safe and healthy, and put food on the table?*
>   David and Sam said Mom "makes sure we eat." Everyone is always helping watch Manny to keep him from getting hurt. Mom always knows where everyone is going. When Sam is outside, he stays where Mom can see him. She had the school district evaluate Manny, and he will receive help with speech.
> 3. *How is Mom nice?*
>   She lets us have dessert and treats after dinner and gives us stuff like toys and clothes. She gives hugs and says, "I love you."
> 4. *Activities?*
>   Mom signed David up for a movie making class. Sam starts baseball next week.
>
> I would like to start having these kinds of conversations with all of you together.

I'm looking forward to our next step which is to build a solid safety plan and move toward Art getting to be with the kids unsupervised. I have a safety planning tool I like to use that should help us. At our agency we typically do a gradual increase in unsupervised time and see how the safety plan is working. *Before we can start that unsupervised time, we need to make this plan.*

Please let me know when we can all meet together!

Talk to you soon,

Beth

This process further solidifies the vision, elicits existing supports for that vision, and identifies specific steps to continue to build on those supports. It can help workers move from simply talking with families about problems that need to change to concretely assisting with specific actions that support directions in life that families themselves have identified (e.g., helping Barb apply for a new job, helping everyone pitch in with watching Manny, possibly coming up with funding that might help David in his moviemaking class). This letter had a profound effect on Art. It confirmed for him that Beth was listening to his family and was interested in keeping him involved in the process. Their connection and his involvement were further enhanced when Beth completed a Collaborative Helping map organized by the same overarching question she had asked Barb ("Twenty years from now, what is the story you hope your children will tell about their childhood and your role in it?"). Figure 4.3 shows that map with the vision statement framed in his sons' voices.

One of the challenges of CPS work is the demand to hold multiple stories simultaneously. On the one hand, we have a story here of a caring father with a commitment to helping his sons become respectful and successful men who do not go "down the wrong road." On the other hand, we have a story of a convicted felon with impulse control problems. Rather than getting caught up in trying to sort out what is the "real" story here, we think it is more efficient and effective to connect with people's better selves without losing sight of troubling problems. Here is where the idea of seeing problems as separate from people becomes particularly useful. CPS could move from a job of "protecting children from maltreating parents" to a job of "partnering with parents to jointly protect their children from problems that pull them away from their better intentions and judgment." Here is where writing up

FIGURE 4.3   **ART'S COLLABORATIVE HELPING MAP**

Art's Vision Statement
"When we were growing up, Dad was helpful. He was there for us in times of need and taught us how to be a man and how a woman should be treated. He was there to see us graduate and see us off to college—or supported us in our business decisions. Our dad was a very funny person and loved joking. He was strict with discipline but also helped us learn to stay away from going down the wrong road. He didn't want us to end up behind bars and said 'I've kind of done time for you guys so you don't have to. You don't want to know what it is like being kept away from the ones you love.' He and Mom were there for us first and taught us that family always comes first."

Obstacles *What pulls you away from this vision?*	Supports *What helps you get to this vision?*
• Falling back into Prison Mode • Art's "anger management issues" • Only having one car • Getting overwhelmed and tired • Art misses his extended family and needs their support • Not having a job is hard on Art who likes working and the family needs money • Art said nothing will pull him away as long as he remembers that he's been behind bars before and does not want to go back	• Talking it out helps the most • Pointing out a problem, analyzing it, and then taking a cooling off time if needed • Grandma is helping a lot with the kids • One-on-one time for Art and Barb for a few minutes to talk; when needed they step outside • Meetings with Art's probation officer • Friends who are constantly checking in with Art

Plan
• Continue talking it out and addressing problems right away • Take cooling off period when needed • Mom and Dad to talk alone for a few minutes when needed • Develop and follow safety plan

danger statements in externalizing language becomes particularly effective. It allows us to juxtapose the vision statement with an externalized danger statement and engage people in a conversation that essentially says, "You've said this is important to you and this is an obstacle that gets in the way of that. Given the importance of this vision to you, what do you want to do about that obstacle?" The juxtaposition of vision statements with harm and danger statements leads quite nicely into safety goals and safety plans.

While the supervised visits continued, Beth began working with Art and Barb to develop a safety plan that would support their goal of reunification and ensure that the kids could be safe when eventually left with Art unsupervised. Central to addressing any issues of harm and danger within a family is the development of a detailed, do-able, and fluid safety plan. The best safety plans are created in collaboration with a family and their extended network, with each member having input while simultaneously agreeing to stick to CPS's bottom lines. Constant monitoring of the plan is done through check-ins with the family and others using scaling questions and adapting the plan as problems arise. Beth used an adaptation of a very useful safety planning tool developed by Sonja Parker (in preparation).[3] The completed plan follows.

Family Safety Plan

Family Details:

Consisting of a brief description of the family

Harm and Danger Statements:

Previously listed

Safety Goals:

- Barb, Art, and the children will be reunited safely with no physical or emotional harm to the kids.
- Barb and Art have repeatedly stated that they want to be together as a family, move to unsupervised time, and raise children who are free from physical and emotional abuse.

Safety Actions Already Happening:

- Barb and Art are experiencing better communication with each other.
- David and Art are experiencing better communication with each other.
- Art is learning to take a cooling off period and express his need for it to the family.

- Barb and Art are committed to not using any physical discipline.
- They are using time-outs with the kids, who are responding to them.

Scaling Question:

0–10 if 0 = no safety at all, and 10 = perfectly safe with the safety actions already happening, Art is at a 7, and Barb is at an 8.[4]

Future Safety Actions:

- Barb and Art will increase their safety number by keeping up with their communication with each other and by talking with the kids about their day, school, feelings, etc.
- Barb and Art will do "purposeful check-ins" with the kids by asking questions such as, "Is there anything you need to talk about? Are you worried about anything?"
- Barb and Art will get on the kids' level—both physically and developmentally when talking with them.
- Art will take a walk for 30 minutes or so to cool off when he needs time alone. Art is aware of when these moments are, and he is committed to leaving the situation to take a break.
- Barb and Art both agree that Art getting a job, and Barb getting a new job will lessen the amount of stress in the family and will contribute to safety.

Scaling Question:

0–10 if 0 = no safety at all, and 10 = perfectly safe, what number would you give with the addition of these future safety actions? Barb and Art are both at a 9.

How Will We Know that the Plan Is Being Followed?

- The kids will report good things if the plan is being followed.

What Will Everyone Do If There Are Problems with the Plan?

- The kids will write it on paper and give it to Barb; they will talk to her. She is very confident that the kids will come to her.

What Will Family Members and Safety Network Members Do If the Kids Tell Them that They Are Worried or Scared?

• Grandma will tell Barb. Art's mom will confront him.

Who Will Check In with the Kids and Parents to Make Sure the Plan Is Working?

• Beth will do monthly check-ins with the family, including seeing the kids individually. Beth will also check in by phone twice monthly.

Presenting the Plan to the Children:

• Beth will go over the plan again with David. She will also make it "Sam-friendly" and go over it with him.

This safety planning tool presents a series of categories to be explored with the family and members of their safety network (extended family, friends, and others who have agreed to be part of a team designed to develop and carry out a safety plan. While safety plans may include services (e.g., AA, therapy, parenting education, etc.), the main focus is on specific actions that the involved parties will take to address the categories and questions outlined earlier. Services, in and of themselves, don't keep children safe. In fact, a written safety plan also doesn't keep children safe. What keeps children safe are the concrete actions and behavioral shifts that people make in carrying out a safety plan. You can see a number of such actions in this plan.

The inclusion of harm and danger statements, safety goals and safety plans represent a valuable addition to the often complicated world of CPS. They provide clear structures to help the various parties who are involved keep focused and stay "in the same book," if not necessarily "on the same page." The addition of vision statements and Collaborative Helping maps in which problems are seen as separate from people builds engagement, invites more participation, and further enhances this work. Moving from concrete harm and danger statements to vision statements that highlight caregivers' own hopes and dreams for their family to an examination of the discrepancies between that vision and the danger statements enhances family "buy in" for safety goals and plans.

USING COLLABORATIVE HELPING MAPS IN THE CHANGING WORLD OF HEALTH CARE

Collaborative Helping has the potential to help change the field of home health care. As reform begins to reshape health-care payment systems, the entire ethos of health care, disease, and wellness shifts. Insurers (both public and private) are beginning to move away from structuring payment around disease treatment toward efforts to promote health. This refocusing will be particularly evident for people with chronic health problems who live in difficult circumstances, including those contending with generational poverty and community-based violence. When health plans make it profitable to enhance the wellness of community members, efforts to promote resilience start to become a higher priority. Practical ways of helping people to help themselves becomes an attractive choice. Home-based supportive helping, so common throughout human services, is now up for serious consideration in the redesign of primary health care especially as a way to leverage personal and community assets for people with complex, long-term health challenges. If someone develops a brain aneurysm, he or she should still get to a technically skilled neurosurgeon as fast as possible. However, if that person also experiences some combination of life's more mundane health challenges like obesity, chronic lung disease, depression, or even aging, a collaborative-style of helping may just be what the primary care doctor of the future orders.

We'll begin with a description of how a Collaborative Helping map was used in a particular health-care situation and then examine some of the broader considerations that are emerging. Willie Jones is a 60-year-old African-American man who lives in a poor urban neighborhood and struggles with hypertension, obesity, and alcoholism. When he drinks heavily, his hypertension tends to become worse. Willie's third wife of 5 years is Myra, a 38-year-old White woman who looks much older than her stated age. During the course of their relationship, Willie's medical condition has deteriorated, and Myra has gained a significant amount of weight. Willie presents himself as a "gregarious soul who everybody knows and loves." Myra, on the other hand, is very worried about Willie coming home tipsy late at night and getting mugged. She continually reminds him to "mind his P's and Q's," which he dismisses, saying, "I know the streets and no one needs to worry over me." While the two bicker constantly, it is immediately apparent that they care deeply about each other and their relationship is very important to each of them.

Willie has a Cuban-American home health worker, Ezra, who has been assigned to help him manage his hypertension and obesity and, in a spirit of harm reduction, reduce his drinking. Willie would love to lower his blood pressure and lose some weight but is skeptical about the idea that his drinking is a problem. While Myra continually nags him about his drinking, she also goes to the local liquor store to restock when Willie is running low on beer so that he is not "out of sorts" when he comes home. Upon learning this, Ezra thinks to himself, "Are you kidding me? You want him to cut down his drinking and to make that happen you buy him a twelve-pack?" He feels caught between his inclination to confront Willie on his drinking and Myra on her code-pendency and his desire to do something different, given that confrontation by other helpers in the past has failed miserably. He settles on the use of a Collaborative Helping map, which his manager has been promoting lately and figures, "What the heck, what harm can it do?"

He explains to Willie and Myra that he has this little "gizmo thing" that he'd like to do with them. He pulls out a sheet of paper, draws a horizontal line a third of the way down the paper and a vertical line below that to make a "T," and then writes Hopes, Obstacles, and Supports on the front and Next Steps on the back. Figure 4.4 illustrates Ezra's creation.

FIGURE 4.4   **AN INFORMAL VERSION OF A COLLABORATIVE HELPING MAP**

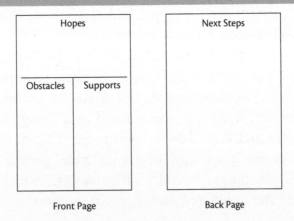

He shows them the piece of paper and explains that he would like to ask them some questions about some of their hopes for their life together, some of the things that could get in the way of those hopes, and some of the things that might contribute to those hopes. He says, "We can try this out and see how far we get." He asks if that would be okay, and they agree.

Ezra then explains that he's worried they might view him as some kind of spy sent by their health-care provider to convince Willie to stop drinking and Myra to stop buying him beers. Willie responds, "Now we're talking." Myra just looks suspicious. Ezra goes on to say that while he's concerned that the combination of hypertension, obesity, and drinking might very well kill Willie and that he would hate to have to show up at his funeral, he's been assured by his boss that he'll get another client and still have a job and so he feels like his own life won't change much regardless of what Willie does. While Myra thinks this is harsh, Willie is beginning to enjoy the conversation. In this process, Ezra has shifted the way in which he is positioned with Willie from someone trying to cure, fix, or change him to someone supporting him in pursuing a desired life in the face of numerous difficulties. This shift in positioning is congruent with both harm reduction and the recovery movement that are both increasingly being incorporated into integrative and collaborative health efforts.

Ezra asks Willie and Myra how many years they think Willie might have left. They both agree three to five years. Willie then adds, "I don't think about that too much. I figure I'll live forever." Myra immediately responds, "Three years tops given his drinking and medical condition." Ezra connects with Willie by saying that while he hopes Willie might actually figure out a way to live forever, he figures it just might not happen. Ezra knows that Willie is a huge fan of Mark Twain and, with this in mind, reminds him of the story of Tom Sawyer sneaking into a funeral held for him and some other boys when it was mistakenly assumed they had drowned in the river. The boys watched their funeral from the balcony of the church. In this vein, he suggests the following to Willie: "Let's assume you check out before Myra and you're up there looking down on Myra talking to her sister Donna (with whom she is very close and who Willie likes a lot) about what the last 5 years of your life together was like. What would you hope she might say?" He asks Myra a similar set of questions and then works with them to craft an informal "obituary" that might come out of Myra's conversation with Donna.

> Willie's health got worse and that was hard, but we had some good times in our last years. I realized again why I fell in love with him in the first place. Donna, you always teased me about taking up with him and he could be really annoying at times. But he was a good man. He always brought light into people's lives and he brought a lot of joy into mine. I realized that I was always fussing at him 'cause he was so damn ornery, but God bless, I miss him. I miss his jokes, the funny way he put things and his general approach to life. You know he'd shoot me if he heard me say this, but while he always presented himself as a jokester who was never serious, talking to children could bring him to tears. He was a gentle and sensitive soul.

At this point, Ezra had to leave, but suggested that they continue doing this "gizmo thing" next time he came back.

Ezra typed up the "obituary" and shared it with Willie and Myra at his next visit. Myra thought it was morbid, but Willie kind of enjoyed it. Ezra asked Willie what he liked about that obituary and what it said about the man he hoped people would remember. Willie read it again, thought a moment, and then said to Myra, "Aw Puddin', I ain't gonna shoot you. Then I'd miss listening to you tell Donna how much you loved me." Myra began to tear up and replied, "You ain't called me Puddin' in years." Ezra asked Myra if she had any pet names she hadn't called Willie in some time and she quickly responded, "Yes, but you're not going to hear them. That's for him to find out tonight after you leave." Willie smiled mischievously and said, "I like this young man. Too many young people lack respect these days." Ezra responded that he appreciated the opportunity this job gave him to learn from his elders. In that context, their relationship continued to shift from Ezra trying to rehabilitate Willie to Ezra learning from him. This relational shift allowed the rest of the conversation to proceed as it did.

Ezra came back to the obituary and asked Willie what he liked about it and how he would like to be remembered after his passing. Willie responded,

> I liked the part about good times and bringing light and joy into people's lives. Life is hard and you have to make the best of it for both yourself and those around you. I'm always trying to pick

people up and help them along on a crappy day. The folks here in my neighborhood, we've all been dealt a lousy hand and sometimes it just makes me so mad. Maybe that's why I get so ornery. But mainly it breaks my heart. You know the streets can be mean and so I don't show that heartbreak so much, but it's still there. I mainly just try to laugh and help people get through another day.

As they sat around the kitchen table, Ezra jotted down a version of that statement on his informal Collaborative Helping map, read it back to Willie and Myra, and asked them what was important about that for them. He also shared how he had been moved in listening to them and how their telling of this story impacted him. Referring back to the vision at the top of the page, Ezra asked about supports and obstacles. Willie described supports as "the highlights of life—the things you strive for" and laid out a number of things. He described obstacles as "the struggles of life—the crap that comes up and drags you down" and also laid out a number of things. Ezra jotted this all down, summarizing what he had heard from Willie, and then, turning the sheet over, asked Willie and Myra how things in the highlights of life category might help with the struggles of life category and wrote that down in the next steps section. He pulled out his cell phone, took a photo of it and sent it to them. Figure 4.5 shows a typed version of the informal map they completed.

This map is just a starting point, but an important one. Its use by Ezra has helped Willie consider his diet and alcohol consumption and lays a foundation for future work. As we look at this map, a number of important considerations emerge. This situation moves from a small medical problem (hypertension, obesity, and substance misuse) to a larger existential problem (how Willie wants to be remembered in his obituary and what he needs to do to increase the chances of that happening). This expansion of medical ailments from their narrow biomedical to broader psychosocial contexts is at the heart of innovations in health care. Collaborative Helping maps provide one way to concretely support this shift. When specific health-care concerns can be framed in the context of larger life concerns, they become more immediately relevant and more amenable to helping efforts. The crucial question here is how helping efforts address what is most relevant to the people we serve. Collaborative Helping maps provide one way to make that important transition.

FIGURE 4.5   WILLIE'S COLLABORATIVE HELPING MAP

Willie's Hopes

I am all about bringing light and joy into people's lives. Life is hard and you have to make the best of it for both yourself and those around you. I'm always trying to pick people up and help them along on a crappy day. The folks here in my neighborhood, we've all been dealt a lousy hand and sometimes it just makes me so mad, but mainly it breaks my heart. The streets can be mean and so I don't show that heartbreak so much. I mainly just try to laugh and help people get through another day, and I really love Myra and want our remaining time to be good.

Obstacles The Struggles of Life	Supports The Highlights of Life
My hypertension wants to kill before I can earn back Myra's love. I get tired of being joyful and want to just zone out. So I drink and then often feel lousy and then we fight. Myra starts worrying about me and nagging me and treats me like a little kid, and I get really ornery and maybe even act like a little kid and that probably gets her worrying more and we just quit talking. Being poor and Black in a country that doesn't give a crap about people in our neighborhood. It pisses me off and I snap at Myra and folks in my neighborhood rather than the system that messes with all of us here.	The love I have for this neighborhood. The love I have for this woman and my worries about her health. Her love for me. Our shared desire to have a good life amid all this crap. My total unwillingness to submit to a system designed to put us down and ignore the fact that it is doing that.

Next Steps

Commitments

I want to be around for this neighborhood because it needs me.
I want to be around for this woman because I love her.

Plan

In order for me to be around for this neighborhood and this woman, I will consider how my eating and drinking messes with that.

CURRENT AND POTENTIAL USES FOR COLLABORATIVE HELPING MAPS

We have explored some of the different ways in which the Collaborative Helping maps have been used. They provide both a structured way to help people think their way through a variety of complex situations and a vehicle for collaborative conversations about challenging issues. In each of these situations, helpers began by building a relationship and then eliciting a vision of people's own hopes for their lives. Subsequent helping efforts assisted them in drawing on their own resources to address potholes on the road to their hopes rather than change becoming a helper-directed process, which could be experienced by them as being operated on rather than worked with.

These maps are pretty simple and many aspects of them have been around for some time. However, we want to highlight several important points that we hope have emerged throughout the various examples. Beginning with a focus on possibilities rather than problems is a very powerful step that enhances engagement, helps to align purposes, sets direction, and builds momentum. Vision provides direction and inspiration, making helping efforts more efficient and effective. Recasting problems as obstacles to preferred directions in life helps us focus on the challenges that are most relevant to be addressed now and narrows our scope down to the most important issues to take up. Viewing obstacles as externalized problems (e.g., thinking about problems as separate from people and people as being in an ongoing and modifiable relationship with those problems rather than being a problem or having a problem) minimizes shame and blame and gives people more maneuverability in addressing those problems. Recasting supports as contributors to preferred directions in life helps us identify supports in a way that is immediately relevant and meaningful to persons involved. Viewing supports as practices in life backed up by intentions, values and beliefs, hopes and dreams, and commitments in life rather than simply individual characteristics leads to richer conversations and helps people build on and further cultivate the supports available to them. The development of a plan that draws on supports to address obstacles and leads to a concrete consideration of "Who will do what, when, and with whom?" takes people to articulated action steps that can hold all involved parties accountable.

Finally, grounding this map in inquiry is very useful. The move from corrective instruction to facilitative inquiry powerfully shifts helping relationships and how helpers and those being helped are positioned with each other. That shift in relational positioning supports the enactment of different life stories and opens up new possibilities for people.

NOTES

1. Madsen's (2007a) book *Collaborative Therapy with Multi-Stressed Families* has chapters on assessment and treatment planning, which gives examples of generic formats for clinical paperwork, including assessments, treatment plans, quarterly reviews, and termination/consolidation summaries.
2. The specifics of breaking this broad question down into a series of questions that become easier to answer are examined further in Chapter 5.
3. Readers interested in learning more about this safety planning tool, and its various uses, can go to www.spconsultancy.au.com.
4. Beth has commented that she usually doesn't write her scaling number on the plan because it is the family's plan. However, she does discuss her rating with the family and, if the respective numbers are too far apart, will work to figure out specifically what needs to happen to bring them closer together.

CHAPTER 5

Engaging People to Envision New Lives

The last two chapters highlighted a simple map intended to help frontline workers think their way through messy situations and to provide a clear framework to organize conversations with people about difficult and challenging issues. These next two chapters move from a broad view of helping efforts overall to a more particular focus on engagement and visioning in this chapter and different ways of talking with people about problems and strengths in the next chapter. The first part of this chapter outlines concrete ways to engage people in helping efforts. The second part highlights questions to help people envision desired futures or preferred ways of coping in a difficult present. And the third part examines ways to accomplish this combined process in challenging situations.

ENGAGEMENT—WHO ARE YOU AND WHAT IS IMPORTANT TO YOU?

In their wonderful book about wraparound, *Everything Is Normal Until Proven Otherwise*, Karl Dennis and Ira Lourie (2006, p. 39) begin a chapter with the following paragraph:

> Does your resume include the fact that you are cranky when you get up in the morning? Does it admit that when you are under pressures, you don't perform as well as you do at other times? Of course not! But don't we do this to young people all the time? The human service agency is the only place where we create resumes for children and youth that only focus on their weaknesses! That's not very fair, is it?

No, it's not. But we seem to work in a business where our initial focus is almost always on problems, sickness, and dysfunction. That's the way payer systems and public bureaucracies are set up. But if we believe that people are more than the sum of problems in their lives, it is useful to initially get to know them outside of those problems. Although we are often required to include "presenting problems" in an intake process, we can still take the opportunity to begin our initial meetings with people around the question of "Who are you and what is important to you?" That's an organizing question to hold in our heads. It's probably too big of a question to ask in such an abstract way, so let's narrow this down.

We can begin by asking people if it would be okay to get to know them outside the immediate concerns or problems that brought them to us. If they agree (which usually happens), we can ask about how they spend their time, what they like to do, and what makes getting up in the morning worthwhile for them. Throughout this process, we can be on the lookout for small instances of competence (moments of resourcefulness), connection (moments where people feel connected to and supported by others), and hope (moments where people have a glimpse that things could be better). We think people's experiences of competence, connection, and hope build a foundation for the development of better lives. These instances are often very small and easy to miss. The trick is to notice them and find ways to expand on them. Experiences of competence, connection, and hope provide a foundation to develop a vision of preferred directions in life that can guide helping efforts.

As an example of this, let's take a look at how Bill often starts meetings with parents and "problematic" children. Usually I'll start by asking if it would be okay to ask the parents some questions to introduce (in this example) their son to me. Assuming they agree, which generally happens, I ask them what I might have come to respect and appreciate about their son if I had known him for 5 years instead of just 5 minutes. I collect a series of descriptors (that often come with qualifying remarks like "he's got brains, if only he'd use them") and highlight the first part ("he's got brains, and what else?") while letting the latter part drop off. When I have an extensive list, I feed it back to the son, ask him if he recognizes himself in that description, and ask him in a conversational way how some of his friends might similarly describe him. I'll usually summarize this combined list and say to the parents something along the lines of, "I understand there have also been some hard things going on and I don't want to lose sight of that, but how have you raised a guy with all these great qualities (listing them out)?" I'll then ask about what they are proud of in their family and what makes that important to them. Marcia Sheinberg and Peter Fraenkel (2001) have described such a process as eliciting stories of pride before stories of shame. Beginning in this way helps both helpers and families realize that people are not simply a collection of problems. Acknowledging strengths and resources also opens space for a more honest and less defensive examination of difficulties.

We see this approach as more than a simple call to focus on the positives. While a strength-based style of engagement is often seen as emphasizing the affirmative, there is more to it than that. Even though the weight of problems may drag us down, hold us back, and even feel like a kind of oppression, people do not easily surrender. Our tendency to resist oppression is part of being human. While words like these are probably more familiar in a context of social justice and human rights, they are also becoming increasingly more relevant as a changed way of thinking about health and well-being. For example, recovery models, a significant trend in health and human services that was introduced in Chapter 1, view helping as a process of enabling people to "get their lives back" with a shift from symptom reduction to enhancing functioning, resilience, and adaptation (Gehart, 2012a, b).

Engaging people can begin by tapping into the desire for a better life and yearning for some greater purpose. Froma Walsh (2010) has offered an expanded view of spirituality as connecting to something larger than oneself. Thinking along these lines, engaging people in a helping relationship is a process of connecting with whatever is important and perhaps even sacred to them. In response to an introductory question of "What makes getting up in the morning worthwhile for you?" a heavily tattooed ex-gang member replies, "The ceramic cast of my infant son's footprint." He goes on to tell a very personal story of how the birth of his son became a turning point resulting in rejection of gang life and a connection to a larger purpose. He says that he's never told that story to anyone before. We can see how such a story shared between a person and a helper can set the stage for future work together. This and other examples of exchanges between helpers and people served are just that, examples. The words are not intended as lines to be used, but instead are samples to illustrate some of the many ways helpers can put a spirit of respect, connection, curiosity, and hope into practice on a routine basis.

VISION—WHERE WOULD YOU LIKE TO BE HEADED IN YOUR LIFE?

In Chapter 3, we discussed the usefulness of organizing collaborative work around a proactive vision of possibilities. This could be a vision of hopes for the future that can provide inspiration and direction for people. It could also be a vision of preferred ways of coping in a difficult present that help people keep their eyes on the prize. A proactive vision is not simply a shift from focusing on problems to focusing on possibilities but an acknowledgment of problems in life along with a focus on desired lives in the face of those difficulties. Let's look at some actual ways to help people develop, elaborate on, and sustain their vision for their lives.

One way to begin these kinds of conversations comes from solution-focused approaches (Berg, 1994; de Shazer, 1985) with the miracle question.

> Suppose one night there is a miracle while you are sleeping and the problem that brought you here is solved. What do you suppose you will notice different the next morning that will tell you that the problem is solved? (Berg, 1994, p. 97)

Often, this question yields a response somewhere along the lines of "I have no idea. . . ." But if we are patient and gently persistent (e.g., "What small things might you first notice?") and ask for details from multiple perspectives (e.g., "And then what would happen . . . and then what . . . and after that, what? And what might your partner, daughter, mother, etc. notice?"), we often are able to trace out a path from the present to this future vision. Another way of approaching that question is to ask people some version of the following questions.

> If we were at the end of our work together rather than the beginning and you were looking back and feeling really good about what you had accomplished in this time, what would be different in your life? How would you know it? Concretely, what would be different in your life together? If we had a YouTube video of you now and another at the end of our work together, what differences would we see?

A similar version of this inquiry to elicit vision statements in a CPS context that was highlighted in the last chapter is "Twenty years from now, what is the story you'd hope your kids would tell about their childhood and your role as their parent in it?" While this has been a powerful question in that context, we can't simply ask it as outlined here and expect people to come up with a comprehensive answer. It has to be adapted to the particularities of different situations and framed in a way that makes it easier to consider. We can ask caregivers what they would like their children to be saying about their upbringing when they are adults. "What story do you prefer to have about your family? What story do you want your kids to tell about their childhood and what it was like for them? When your kids are 25 years old, and someone asks them about their upbringing, how do you hope they will describe you as their parent?" We can ask parents to finish this sentence in their children's voices as if their children are now adults: "When I was growing up my mother was or my father was. . . ."

This vision question is a big question for people if they haven't thought through it. We can facilitate these discussions by asking parents to talk about the important components of a childhood: "In your opinion, what makes up a good childhood? What categories (family, friends, education, religion, activities, character, work, nurturing, discipline, etc.) do you want to make sure you are paying attention to for your kids? Is there something you would wish to improve on in comparison to your own upbringing? Is there something you want to give your kids that you didn't receive? Is there something you received that you hope to pass down to your kids?" Beth Root (Root and Madsen, 2013), who uses these questions on a regular basis, has emphasized the importance of making sure that the issues that brought a family into contact with CPS are included in this conversation.

> For example, if there are safety issues around physical abuse, I might ask, "And how do you want to be disciplining them? If they were 25 and somebody asked them what did your mom do for discipline or how did your dad handle it when you acted out, what would you hope they might say?" And then you can get a comment on that: "Well, I don't want to be using physical discipline. I actually don't think it's right. That was a mistake that I did that. I'd rather be using time-outs or taking away privileges." So that can go right into the vision statement.

Not surprisingly, the answers to these questions are usually totally incongruent with the problems that bring us to a family's door and provide a solid foundation for examining the obstacles that stand in the way of that vision as well as the supports that might contribute to achieving that vision.

Sometimes people have trouble envisioning alternative futures. At these times, questions from appreciative inquiry may be useful. Appreciative inquiry is an approach to organizational consultation that draws on the best of "what is" to envision "what might be" and develop "what will be" (Cooperrider, et al., 2000). Examples of questions from appreciative inquiry in a helping context might include:

- Everyone has days when they are "off," when they are not "at their best." As you might guess, I am going to need to ask you about that in a bit. But, before I do, can I ask you a little bit about when you are "on," when you are "at your best" as a parent?
- Can you think of a particular moment when you felt good about yourself as a parent? What was happening? What were you doing? How were your children responding?
- As you think about that moment, what did you particularly value or appreciate about what you did and how you did it? What makes that important to you? What might that say about your hopes and dreams for yourself as a parent?
- Imagine it is a year from now and those things you appreciate about yourself as a parent in your best moments were showing up more and more. How would you know it? Concretely, what would be happening? If we had a YouTube video of you in this future moment, what would we see on it? What difference would this make for you and your family?

These are sample questions and it is important to ask them as part of a back-and-forth conversation in which each answer shapes the next question rather than as a script to be followed. However, this can be a very powerful process. Because the vision that comes out of these questions is based on actual moments and grounded in real experience and history, it is both achievable and meaningful for people.

At times, the invitation to focus on "best moments" can feel disqualifying of the pain and difficulty in people's lives. In such situations, questions developed by Robert Kegan and Lisa Laskow Lahey (2000) can be useful to use people's complaints to elicit hopes and commitments. The following questions highlight an example with a mother complaining about her daughter:

- What is your biggest complaint about your relationship with your daughter (making sure to move a complaint about the daughter to a complaint about their relationship)?
- What would you like to see instead?
- If your complaint and your hope for something different were somehow a message about what you really care about, what is important to you, what you value, what might that message be? (It can be helpful to put the answer in the frame of "I am committed to the value or importance of _____ in our relationship.")
- If your relationship with your daughter were grounded in those commitments, concretely how would we know it? What would be different between you?
- Would that be important to you and why? How might that change your relationship with your daughter?

Throughout these questions it's important to keep a focus on what the mother can do differently rather than simply a focus on what the mother expects her daughter to do differently. Almost all of us have had relationship difficulties at some point in our life and all too often it is apparent what the easiest solution would be—the other person needs to change. Unfortunately, changing other people is something over which we have little control. Staying focused on what we can change in our own lives can be frustrating, but it is probably more productive. Returning now to the visioning questions, this combination of appreciative inquiry questions and complaint to commitment questions gives us the flexibility to meet people where they are at presently in order to draw on their best moments and/or greatest frustrations to envision possibilities.

Once we have the beginnings of a vision, we can expand on it by building a foundation of motivation (Why is this vision important to you?), resourcefulness (When have you been able to bring bits of this vision into your life?), and community (Who in your life appreciates this vision and has supported you or might support you in the future in realizing it?). These questions can solidify visions and are ones that we can come back to repeatedly to help people stay connected to their vision and sense of purpose in life.

To complete this section on visioning, let's look at the work of Sonja Parker (2013), who has developed a very useful visual tool called the "Future House." We want to highlight this because it expands our repertoire from just talking to engaging in a concrete activity with people.[1] This tool was originally designed to help parents or caregivers involved with CPS. However, we have found it very useful across a wide variety of situations and it can be done with both parents and children, alone or together. We'll focus the discussion here on how it has been used in CPS situations with a parent. Figure 5.1 highlights the various parts of the Future House.

The process begins with a worker sitting down alongside a parent and drawing a house on a large sheet of paper. We can then say something along the lines of "The purpose of this project is to help me and other professionals get a better sense of your hopes for your children and how you want to take care of them." That leads easily into the questions such as the ones listed inside the house in Figure 5.1 for purposes of illustration. Parents' responses to such questions can be written or drawn

FIGURE 5.1   **THE FUTURE HOUSE**

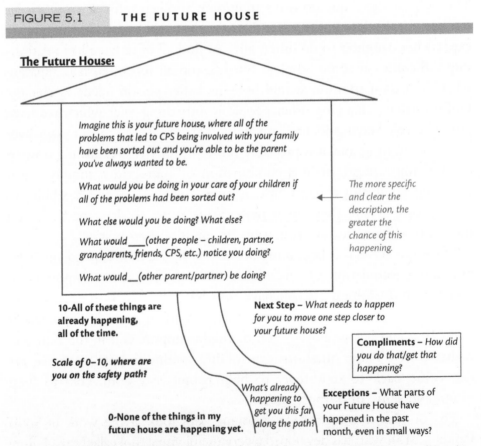

Used with the permission of Sonja Parker. From *The Future House Tool: Involving Parents and Caregivers in the Safety Planning Process* (2013).

by them or the worker, based on their preference. In this process, it is important to get concrete details of the future vision. Parker (2013) cites solution-focused research that shows that the more specific and detailed people's descriptions are of what they would be doing in the future, the more likely it is that they will actually do this. It is also useful to ask parents questions from other people's points of view (such as the fourth question inside the house in Figure 5.1), always keeping a focus on what a parent concretely would be doing in his or her care of children so that CPS involvement is not needed. As we've emphasized throughout this book, the spirit with which workers approach this process is paramount. This tool is based on two key implicit assumptions:

1. We believe that future safety is possible for their children.
2. We believe that family members also want a safe future for their children.

It is important to ask these questions in ways that communicate these assumptions and leave people feeling they are in a respectful conversation rather than an interrogation. As mentioned earlier, once we have a Future House vision, we can ask questions about motivation, resourcefulness, and community. (Why is this in particular important to you? When have there been times when some of what you've described here has already been happening, even if it's just in small ways? Who else might appreciate your Future House and stand with you in getting to it?) The next part of the Future House is the safety path, which asks a parent to identify how much of this preferred future is already happening. The safety path is the curved path in Figure 5.1 from the bottom of the page to the house. It provides a visual representation of a scaling question (On a scale of 0 where none of what you've described in your Future House is happening yet to 10 where all of what you're describing is already happening, where would you say you're currently at?). Once people have located themselves on the safety path (often with a line or a stick figure), we can inquire further about how they've gotten as far along as they have (even in small ways) and what would be the next action to move one step closer to their Future House. This becomes a way of recording what is already happening in order to both acknowledge and build on that and invites parents to describe what they see as the next steps in working toward a preferred safe future for their children. When completed, we can ask parents with whom they might be willing to share their Future House. Having this project witnessed by someone important to the parents can be very powerful. The Future House also provides a touchstone that we can revisit over time to inquire about how they've moved forward, when that has happened, and what support they might need if they've slipped back. This is a quick overview of a more nuanced tool, but one we wanted to highlight because of its visual nature and its congruency with Collaborative Helping. Literally drawing out a Future House offers a different way to explore vision with people, and the safety path provides a way to identify both obstacles and supports on that path, leading to a clear and detailed process for moving forward. From here, let's move into challenges that can develop when we are engaging people to envision preferred directions in life.

ENGAGEMENT DIFFICULTIES

Our efforts to engage reluctant individuals and families are influenced by our beliefs about motivation, resistance, and "denial," and there are a number of ways to rethink commonly held assumptions. Motivational interviewing has emphasized the importance of entering into a person's worldview to examine the discrepancy between future goals and current behavior. Miller and Rollnick (2013) stress that motivational interviewing is not a set of techniques but rather an interpersonal style for building motivation for change and strengthening people's commitment to change. They highlight four general principles behind motivational interviewing that include:

1. **Express empathy**—See the world through the eyes of people served.
2. **Develop discrepancy**—Help people examine the gap between future goals and current behavior.
3. **Roll with resistance**—Help people examine new perspectives, but don't impose new ways of thinking on them.
4. **Support self-efficacy**—Support people in the belief that change is possible.

Solution-focused therapy has distinguished between customer, complainant, and visitor relationships and offered strategies for responding to each (Berg, 1991, 1994; Berg & Miller, 1992; de Shazer, 1988). Customer relationships are those in which a complaint or goal has been jointly identified by people and helpers and where people see themselves as part of the solution and are willing to do something about the situation. Complainant relationships are those in which people see a significant problem but don't believe they have any control or influence over the situation and are unable to do something about it. Visitor relationships are those in which people do not believe that what others are identifying as a problem is particularly concerning and as a result are not willing to take action to address it. In each of these situations, it is important to keep in mind the solution-focused emphasis on these situations as descriptions of helping relationships rather than descriptions of personal characteristics. Engagement or reluctance to engage is always an interactional process. This contention may seem like a stretch at times, particularly when workers find themselves stymied in their desire to be helpful. However, it is useful to assist us in staying focused on our own actions as a factor over which we have some control. We will pull together ideas from motivational interviewing and solution-focused approaches with ideas about responding to situations in which people come to hold a "No Problem Stance"—this is not a problem and I don't need to address it—and a "No Control Stance"—this is a problem, but I have no control over it and can't address it (Madsen, 1992, 2007a).

A No Problem Stance often develops in situations where there is substance abuse, violence, physical abuse, sexual abuse, neglect, and other situations characterized by "denial." We put the word denial in quotation marks here to highlight it as a label that helpers are assigning to the situation and to help us view it as an interactional process rather than an individual characteristic. In these situations, helpers can end up trying to get people to see that a problem exists and engage in a struggle to get the person to acknowledge or agree with how they see things. People who hold a No Problem Stance are likely to respond with counterarguments that rigidify that stance and threaten the helping relationship. Over time, these interactions can take on a life of their own and become a situation in which each party's response invites a counterresponse from the other. This can be represented as shown in Figure 5.2.

Helpers' arguments for the need for change may invite a person to respond by defending the status quo. At the same time, that person's arguments that "It's really not that big a deal; I don't see what you are so worried about," invites the helper to more strongly confront that stance.

FIGURE 5.2   INTERACTIONS AROUND A NO PROBLEM STANCE

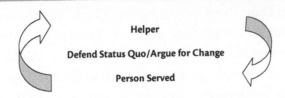

As these interactions take on a life of their own, we can shift from think-ing about "people doing the pattern" to the "pattern doing the people." Paradoxically, interactional patterns that develop around a No Problem Stance may inadvertently rigidify that stance and further impede helping efforts. A No Problem Stance and the interactions that occur around it can be seen as an obstacle that hinders people from more effectively addressing problems. We can shift from seeing the person as the problem to viewing the stance as the problem. As helpers respond to these stances, the interactions that develop further constrain attempts to address the problems.

A No Control Stance often manifests itself when parents call about out-of-control youths (mental illness, substance misuse, violence, and high-risk situations that include suicidal behavior, running away, risky sexual behavior, etc.) or when spouses call about their partner's sub-stance misuse, gambling, or other problematic behavior. In these situa-tions, people seeking help are often focused on trying to help someone else change (despite that person's lack of interest in change) instead of focusing on changes that could be made in their own life. Attempting to help people in these situations can be frustrating and people can often become labeled as "passive," an "enabler," or "codependent." In this situation, helpers can fall into attempting to convince people that they can do something about the problem and they in turn can experience the helper's actions as "minimizing" the magnitude of their difficulties and respond with arguments for why change is not possible. The inter-actional patterns that develop around a No Control Stance can inadver-tently rigidify that stance. Figure 5.3 portrays this pattern.

Again, this interactional pattern can rigidify a No Control Stance. As people minimize the degree of control they have over a situation, they find themselves increasingly drawn into despair and a sense of lack of control, which limits their ability to address the problem.

FIGURE 5.3	INTERACTIONS AROUND A NO CONTROL STANCE

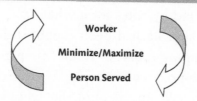

Worker
Minimize/Maximize
Person Served

Each of these situations presents helpers with a dilemma. If we confront a No Problem Stance or a No Control Stance, we run the risk of falling into a "defend the status quo/argue for change sequence" or a "minimize/maximize sequence" that inadvertently rigidifies that stance. If we don't confront that stance, we run the risk of colluding with it. Either choice is problematic, so what are we to do?

Let's explore alternatives to this dilemma. We can approach both these situations (No Problem Stance and No Control Stance) with two important shifts in practice. The first shift is moving from what causes the stance (e.g., Why are people holding a No Problem Stance or a No Control Stance?) to what constrains people from more effectively addressing the problem. The second shift is moving from a role in which helpers confront that stance to one in which helpers invite people to critically reflect on that stance (Jenkins, 1990). This second shift is perhaps the more important one because as motivational interviewing has suggested, it is the person's job to resolve ambivalence about change and the helper's job to ask questions that help the person reflect on his or her situation. The next sections offer concrete suggestions to accomplish this in ways that both honor and acknowledge a problematic stance while opening possibilities for change.

ENGAGING A YOUTH WITH A NO PROBLEM STANCE

We'll illustrate this with a story of a youth Bill worked with some years ago. Vinny is a 17-year-old Italian-American young man who dropped out of high school to become a guitarist in a punk rock band. According to Vinny, he and his band are on the verge of signing a major record contract after which he will be "set for life." He lives with his parents in a suburban neighborhood where finding practice space for a punk band can be difficult. Vinny and his band had worked out a deal with the drummer's family to let them practice in their basement. I had been meeting with Vinny and his folks for a while, and one evening, his parents brought him in after he had been caught stealing alcohol from the drummer's father's liquor cabinet. While his parents were very upset about this, Vinny's response was simply, "Hey, what's the problem? If he didn't want us to take his alcohol, he would have locked it up." They asked if I would talk with him about this situation and I agreed with the proviso that we all would have a conversation afterward. My conversation with Vinny was guided by four principles that I have often used in such situations:

1. **First do no harm**—Avoid interactions that are likely to rigidify problematic stances.
2. **Connection before correction**—First connect with people's intentions, hopes, values, and preferred view of self.
3. **Mind the gap**—Elicit and examine discrepancies between people's intentions, hopes, values, and preferred view of self and the current effects of their actions.
4. **Grow the exception into a plan for change**—Build on this exception to a No Problem Stance to develop an agreed-upon focus for shared work.

First Do No Harm

Recognizing a No Problem Stance and the potential for an interaction that would further rigidify that stance, I suppressed my initial response of "Are you freaking kidding me? You have got to take some responsibility," and instead commented, "Vinny, that's an interesting response. How have others responded? What did the father say to you? What did your friend the drummer say and think about this? What did your band mates say and think about this? What did your parents say and think about this? What do you think about these various responses to this situation?" Getting a better sense of the terrain of responses allowed me to more carefully think about how I would want to weigh in on this and how I might avoid a "defend the status quo/argue for change" sequence (as highlighted back in Figure 5.2) that would probably rigidify Vinny's No Problem Stance. I wanted to enter our conversation in a way that might lead to a different outcome.

Connection Before Correction

I began by asking Vinny a number of questions like, "What was going on? What was happening? When you took the alcohol, what was your intention? What were you looking to accomplish, etc.?" He told me a story of how there was a party coming up and he was in charge of getting the alcohol for the party. He had a fake ID that had been confiscated in a liquor store 2 weeks ago and the local drunk they often relied on to score alcohol at their back-up liquor store was curiously missing in action. Vinny described himself as being at his wit's end. He knew that people were counting on him to come up with the alcohol and he basically said, "What choices did I have? I'm a man of my word and I deliver on my promises. That is what responsibility is all about." The idea of an under-age minor stealing alcohol as an example of responsibility was a bit of a stretch for me, but holding to the principle of "connection before correction," I bit my tongue (for the time being) and continued on in the conversation. (Here's a way of thinking about this that might help you as the reader also stay in the spirit of this process. Have you ever shown up at a potluck without a dish to contribute? It can be embarrassing because we all want to contribute. We are not endorsing Vinny's actions here; we are simply entering into his internal logic to more effectively invite him to reflect on the effects of his actions and open possibilities for other responses to emerge on his part.) In that context, I could connect with Vinny's experience that people were counting on him and he needed to deliver in order to honor and acknowledge this intention as a foundation from which to more effectively challenge his actions. I asked Vinny a number of questions about this idea of him being a man people counted on: what he liked about that view of him, what was important about it to him, and what values and beliefs it tapped into. This appreciation of his best intentions and preferred view of self provided a foundation to move on to the next step of examining the discrepancy between that preferred view of self and the actual effects of his actions.

Mind the Gap

This principle comes from an exhortation often heard in the London Underground referring to the need to attend to the gap between subway cars and the station platform. Similarly, we can help people notice and examine the gap between their intentions and preferred view of self and the actual effects of their actions. In that context, I said to Vinny, "You know, on the one hand I'm listening to you and I get the importance of you being a man of your word, a man of principle, a man who is responsible. On the other hand, I'm holding this story of a man whose actions have resulted in his band now being without a practice space on the eve of an important gig that could make a huge difference for your band's future and how that kind of puts your band up the creek. I'm struggling with this a bit. How do you put those two things together?" That question led to the following exchange:

Vinny: Yeah, that's pretty screwed up. I left my band high and dry in this and I don't feel good about that.

Bill: You know, Vinny, a lot of guys would have a hard time copping to that. It'd be much easier to simply blow it off and say you were unjustly accused. And yet here you are saying, "Yeah, I did that and it screwed things up for my band." What does it tell you about yourself that you are able to acknowledge this and not blow it off?

Vinny: Well, it tells me that, as I said, I'm a man of my word and it's important to face facts.

Do you notice how Vinny's statements here are a bit of an exception to the prevailing stance of "my actions are not a problem?" It's a small start (he is not acknowledging his stealing as a problem), but it is a start. The art here is honoring his intentions enough to allow him to sit with the discomfort of that discrepancy and discomforting him enough in that discrepancy that he may decide to take action to resolve it. His acknowledgment of some of the effects of his actions is a starting point from which we can begin to build an alternative story and responses to the situation.

Grow the Exception into a Plan for Change

As a follow-up to this previous exchange, I asked Vinny, "As a man of your word, what do you want to do to make this up to your band?" We explored this idea and Vinny decided to go to the father whose alcohol he had stolen and say to him, "Look, man, I screwed up and I am really sorry about what I did. I should not have stolen your alcohol and I will pay you back for it. But this is my screw-up. Please don't punish my band. If I agree not to show up, can my band still rehearse in your basement?" The father appreciated this response, thought it showed integrity, and allowed the band to practice there as long as Vinny agreed not to set foot in his house. A month later, Vinny's band had performed at a couple gigs that served as practice sessions for Vinny. The drummer spoke to his father, saying, "You know Dad, we're not doing so well without Vinny having a chance to practice with us." The father in response called up Vinny and said, "You know, Vinny, you've held true to your word and so here's the deal. When you have finished paying me off for the alcohol, you can come back and practice in my basement with the band, but know this. If you ever steal alcohol from me again, I will break your fingers." (While this was probably not a serious threat, the father was someone from whom you did not take such statements lightly.) Vinny agreed and went on to play with his band. While they never received the breakthrough recording contract, he has continued to enjoy playing music and holds a leadership position in the band.

While there were some specific interactions that contributed to Vinny's shift in all of this, it is important to strike a balance between the particular words that were said to Vinny and the spirit behind them. The words were important and opened space for other possibilities to emerge. However, those words as a template to follow without a spirit of respect, connection, curiosity, and hope behind them would ring hollow. Once again, we return to the fundamental importance of the attitude or relational stance with which we approach people in Collaborative Helping.

ENGAGING A WOMAN WITH A NO CONTROL STANCE

Margie is an elderly Polish-American woman struggling with diabetes. She holds a pessimistic view of her future and spends a lot of time bemoaning her fate of dying before her time and never having a chance to live out the dreams she and her husband had to travel to Italy upon retirement. Her husband, Walter, also Polish-American, is a retired salesman who devoted his life to bringing the power of positive thinking into his successful career. He continually encourages Margie to hold a more positive attitude toward her illness and her prospects in life. They are locked into the same kind of minimize/maximize sequence that was highlighted back in Figure 5.3 in which Walter's efforts to help Margie hold a more positive attitude are experienced by her as minimizing the realities of her situation, and Margie's responses to his efforts are experienced by Walter as catastrophizing a life situation that could be changed. A common exchange between them goes as follows:

Walter: Honey, your worries about your medical condition are going to do you in. Sitting around and anticipating your death is not going to help you in any way. You have to get a better attitude about your illness.

Margie: Okay, how's this for a better attitude? My diabetes is going to kill me and our travel dreams, but think of all the money you'll save on the cost of my ticket when you travel without me.

Walter: Honey, if I had taken that attitude in my sales career, we would never have saved enough money to retire and even contemplate our travel plans.

You can imagine Margie's response to Walter and see how they are locked in a sequence in which she perceives his statements as minimizing her situation, which invites her to emphasize how bad things are, and he perceives her as maximizing her horrible predicament, which invites him to reassure her that things would be better if she could just get a better attitude. Unfortunately, this sequence places Margie in a position in which she is continually emphasizing how little influence she has over her medical condition and inadvertently rigidifies a No Control Stance.

This context presents significant problems for Kristen, an outreach nurse who meets with Margie in her home to monitor her diabetes. As part of their time together, Kristen and Margie often sit at the kitchen table, drinking tea, and talking about many different things including her medical condition. The following principles helped Kristen address this situation:

- **First do no harm**—Avoid interactions that may rigidify problematic stances.
- **Connection before correction**—Search for hopes behind complaints.
- **Look for agency**—Examine people's responses to problematic situations and listen for instances that hold self-efficacy or agency.
- **Grow the exception into a plan for change**—Build on exceptions to a No Control Stance to develop an agreed-upon focus for shared work.

First Do No Harm

Kristen knows from experience that pointing out to people who hold a No Control Stance that they might in fact have more influence over their life situation is a fruitless endeavor and likely to rigidify that stance. As a result, she bites her tongue, holds back what she would like to say, and instead asks a number of questions. She asks Margie what it's like to live with Diabetes (thinking of it as a problem separate from Margie) and what effects that situation has on her. In the process, she attempts to develop a deep appreciation for what this situation might be like for Margie and listens with empathy to her story of woe, inquiring about what is particularly problematic about the situation for her.

Connection Before Correction

As Margie complains about the situation, Kristen listens for the hopes behind her complaints. A story emerges of how Margie and Walter always wanted to travel to Italy in their retirement and Margie feels victimized by her medical condition and how it makes such travel plans seemingly impossible. Kristen learns about their hopes for that trip and what made it particularly important to them. Rather than attempt to point out that they still might be able to travel despite Margie's medical condition, she empathizes with her disappointment and asks how she has been coping with it.

Look for Agency

Kristen learns from Margie that she and Walter have been making periodic trips into the North End of Boston (an old Italian section of town) and pretending they were visiting Italy. In this description of her response, Margie is not just a passive victim of her situation, but someone who is actively responding to it. Kristin seeks to learn more about Margie's agency and self-efficacy in the situation. As she asked Margie about what those trips are like, what she likes about them, and the meaning they hold for her, she is looking for active steps that Margie is taking to respond differently. In these small steps, Margie moves from an experience of herself as a person passively victimized by her medical condition to a person actively responding to and coping with it. Kristin expands on this by asking Margie how her life is different when she and Walter are on these outings, how her view of the future is different, and how her life in general feels different.

Grow the Exception into a Plan for Change

You can see how in this situation, Margie is beginning to describe actions that fall outside a sense of having no control over her medical situation. Kristen comments that many people in Margie's situation could be totally captured by Diabetes and wonders how it is that Margie has managed to continue to build a life she prefers for herself in the face of Diabetes' influence. Margie comments that she hadn't realized she was doing that and together they agree to look for ways to build more of a life that she would prefer despite Diabetes' influence. This does not end with "and they lived happily every after." The minimize/maximize sequence between Margie and Walter was still quite embedded and it took them awhile to disengage from that. Margie's medical condition is improving, but she still has setbacks. Kristen's grounding in these principles helped her to engage Margie in a way that stripped away some of the additional constraints to managing her medical condition. We will take up a continuation of their conversation in the next chapter.

Again, we come back to the idea of interactions between helpers and the people they serve as definitional ceremonies. In the course of these interactions, both Vinny and Margie came to experience themselves in some significantly different ways. We have talked about "walking and talking" with an eye toward organizing helping interactions in ways that shift people's experience of self and the stories they come to hold about their lives. These are continued examples of concrete ways to do that. We think the process of walking alongside people and engaging them in ways that open possibilities for a different experience of life has great potential to enhance the effectiveness of helping efforts.

DIFFICULTIES DEVELOPING A VISION

It can be difficult to help people develop a vision in the midst of perpetual crises that leave little room for envisioning alternatives or when they are caught in a life that seems so bleak that hope for the future appears an irrelevant enterprise. We consider each of these situations in turn.

Helping People Envision a Life Outside of Everyday Crises

One of the realities of life for many people in multi-stressed situations is that life can often seem like a progression of unrelenting crises that just need to be endured. There is a deep paradox here. In the face of real and significant crises, if people don't respond to those crises, there may be no future. At the same time, if they don't take time to step out of crisis, they may not escape the tyranny of perpetual crises. While it is vitally important to respond to urgent serious concerns, taking the time to help people momentarily step outside the immediacy of reactive crises helps them better respond to those crises. However, it requires a leap of faith that inviting people to step out of a crisis to reflect rather than simply react will be beneficial in the long run. Let's look at one example of trying to strike that balance.

Manny and Irma are a Puerto Rican couple with an 18-year-old daughter, Nanine, who is struggling with depression, anxiety, self-harm, and substance misuse. She is very reactive to them and they are at their wit's end in trying to figure out how to control her behavior in order to keep her safe. They consult María, a Latina outreach counselor who feels nervous about the enormity of the situation and wonders whether they should be seeing someone from the health center with more credentials and experience. The parents are very clear that they will only see a person who understands their community and the realities of their daily life, and María realizes that she may be their best and perhaps only hope. She is buoyed up by an outside consultant who suggests that what she may lack in learned experience could be more than compensated for in lived experience and who offers to provide ongoing support for her in working with the family. After two meetings devoted to trying to solve immediate and pressing problems, María asks Manny and Irma if it would be okay to step back and take a few minutes to consider their hopes for their daughter's future. They agree (although they find the request a bit strange), and she asks them about their hopes for the daughter they brought to the States from Puerto Rico 10 years ago. María then says, "I know this is kind of an unusual question, but let's assume it's 10 years from now and Nanine is doing okay in her life and is safe. What's the story you would hope she would tell about these last 10 years and your role in helping her to keep herself safe and healthy?" This question helped Manny and Irma to step back from the immediacy of the situation and they each responded with thoughtfulness and tenderness.

María jotted down what they were saying and changed their future tense into three present tense principles:

- We are a stable, loving force and respond calmly when she is out of control.
- We hold strict limits to keep her safe and she knows we care about her and believe in her.
- We are always there for her and we never give up on her.

María asked whether this captured what they had said (it did), suggested that they would probably have a number of opportunities to help Nanine develop her capacity to keep herself safe over the next bit of time, and wondered whether these might be good principles to help guide their responses to the crises in Nanine's life. Manny and Irma felt these principles were very helpful, and María's job shifted from trying to solve vexing problems for the family to helping the parents put these principles into practice in daily life with their daughter.

In this interaction, María probably spent about 10 minutes asking about the parents' hopes for their daughter. While taking this short bit of time in the midst of a crisis can often feel like a stretch, we would suggest that it is a useful investment of time. Their stepping back from the immediacy of the situation, connecting with deeper hopes for their daughter, and reflecting on how best to respond to her in crises helped them to develop a sense of "we can get through this" in responding to her. This situation is also not another happily ever after story. Nanine went on to have a tough couple of years and her parents' abilities to respond to her were often sorely tested, but they did get through it. María's shift to a role of reminding Nanine's parents of the principles they had developed and commending them on their creative implementation of those principles (as well as periodically helping them brainstorm in the process) made her job much more rewarding.

Working With People Who Have Little Hope for the Future

Many workers have had the experience of asking young people, "What do you think your life will look like in 5 years?" only to be met with a rather flat, matter of fact response of "I'll be dead." Not a pretty future and not an auspicious beginning for hopeful work! The reality is that many people on the margins of our society have been beaten down and convinced that their life has no possibilities (and even if it did, they wouldn't deserve it). In that context, inquiring about possible futures may simply add insult to injury and contribute to further demoralization. So, what are other possibilities?

One possibility is to look for what is important and meaningful to someone and try to build on that. Here are some examples of that from an interview with Marianne, director of a community outreach program for marginalized inner city Black and Latino youth, many of whom are gang involved.

What are some of the ways in which you help gang members develop a vision for their life when they don't believe they have a future?

One of the things I try to do is help them envision a hypothetical one. So I might say, "Let's say you have a son or daughter and she is now 5 years old. What do you hope will be happening for that child?" They seem to be able to reach that fairly easily and focus on their cares for someone else. So then I might say, "Now imagine they're 12 and hanging out with some friends who are kind of homieish and kind of gangsterish. How do you feel about that?" And they will start to create for this child the kind of vision they really want for themselves and they will talk about hopes and dreams and eventually I ask them, "What does that mean to you as far as your life? Is that something you wished could have happened in your life?" And many of them will say, "Of course." And I can then take that and break it down into their current daily life: "Okay, now let's say you're able to make some changes in your life and I'm not saying it's possible because everything surrounding you isn't something I can do anything about and maybe isn't something you can do anything about, but what parts of what you just told me are things you might find yourself being able to do?" And any comments about being more conscious about where they're at, how they look, what they can do about their exposure, how they keep their families safe, what might be some things they could do that would move them closer to the goal that they talked about for the hypothetical child. I'm trying to get them to think about themselves as having possibilities. They seem to have a whole bunch of ideas for a child that we can make up, but for themselves it is harder, and so I have to use a step that is once-removed for them to be able to talk about a future because I think they've been so saturated with this idea that they're really not worth much, that I have to take it away from them and have something they can care about and put what they're really hoping for into that being.

Do you have any other examples of this?

> Yeah, another example would be a guy who had to cross multiple neighborhoods in his daily life where wearing colors could probably get him killed. It wouldn't work to talk with him about the importance of keeping himself safe because he didn't care about that. But finding out who or what he did care about and focusing there made a lot of difference. I learned that his girlfriend was really important to him and asked him, "How would it be if some guys rolled up on you and asked, 'Where you from?' and when you answered, they started blasting and you didn't get hit, but your girlfriend did. How would that be?" And he was like, "Damn, man, it's okay if I get hit, but not her, not her." And that opened up space for what he might do differently. He began to dress differently. He avoided looking guys in the eye as they passed by. He put on a pair of glasses so he looked a little bit less thuggish. He wanted to protect her so he always kept her away from the street and he dressed differently and he carried himself differently so he didn't seem like he was banging, in order to protect her. And then, he realized that way of moving through his life worked better for him. He didn't have to always be looking over his shoulder and he began to change how he lived his life. But it started with his love of her because that was important to him.

These two examples highlight the usefulness of initially finding out what is important to people because that may provide something powerful to come back to in attempting to help them step outside a world that increasingly constricts them.

A final example of this comes from a much less dire situation. A school guidance counselor was working with an 8-year-old girl who had been really mean to other girls in her class. Her response when confronted about this was a completely disinterested "I don't care." Her guidance counselor had a strong connection with her and knew that she really loved her old and battered "Dolly," a doll that had been her closest companion for many years. The guidance counselor knew Dolly was important to this girl and engaged her in a conversation about their friendship, what kind of friend she was to Dolly, what Dolly might really like about this girl as her friend, and the impact on the girl herself of her being such a good friend to Dolly. From there, the guidance counselor was able to have a conversation with the girl about what kind of friend she might like to be to other children in her class and what impact that might have on the girl herself. The girl thought other children might appreciate good friends in the same way that Dolly had appreciated her friendship and found it to be in her interest to become that kind of friend with others.

So, what crosscutting themes do you notice in these various stories? We would describe some of the general principles in action here as follows:

- Find something that is important, meaningful, and relevant to a person.
- Build on that to envision possibilities outside what currently seems available to that person.
- Connect those possibilities to relevant areas of the person's current life.
- Examine with them what might be important about building on this and what are some of the ways in which they have already begun to do that.

CONNECTING TO BUILD DESIRED FUTURES

We have repeatedly emphasized the importance of grounding helping work in a spirit of respect, connection, curiosity, and hope. In this chapter, we have highlighted some concrete ways to connect with people as three-dimensional human beings outside of the difficulties in their lives. When we begin with an assumption that people are more than a collection of symptoms, our helping efforts are enhanced. It creates a foundation that allows us to start in a different fashion and build a helping relationship that is much more likely to yield benefits. There is an interesting interplay between engagement and vision. The people we help need to feel a strong enough relational connection with us as helpers to be willing to share their visions for preferred directions in life. And the process of eliciting such vision enhances relationship. The two are intimately connected to each other in so many ways. We trust that real stories told about actual practices of engagement and vision will help you in your own efforts in this combined process, particularly in challenging situations.

▪ NOTE

1. Readers who are interested in learning more about the Future House and getting examples of its use in everyday practice can go to www.spconsultancy.com.au.

CHAPTER 6

Rethinking Problems and Strengths

As we get to know people and work with them to develop a forward-thinking vision to guide shared work, we can also begin the tricky business of talking about obstacles and supports. This chapter rethinks the way we consider problems and strengths and suggests some creative ways to address obstacles and draw on supports.

We have repeatedly stressed relational connection as the heart of helping work. This is especially true in conversations with people about problems in their lives. For example, imagine finding yourself in a situation where you've been assigned to talk to a complete stranger about something that you find uncomfortable, embarrassing, or shameful. You don't know this person and are nervous about how they might treat you. What would you need from them to be willing to talk openly and honestly? How would you want them to relate to you? What would you want them to notice about you? How might they interact that would convince you it would be okay and maybe even helpful to talk with them? The Golden Rule might work here (Treat others the way you would like to be treated). But let's move even further to the Platinum Rule (Treat others the way you think *they* might want to be treated). If we can find ways to talk about problems that minimize the possibility of shame and blame, our work can become much more effective. Using the idea of "externalizing" from narrative approaches that was originally introduced in Chapter 3, we explore ways to accomplish this feat.

Similarly, strengths-based service planning has become somewhat of a cliché in health and human services. Too often the person completing an intake is prompted to list strengths as an addendum (almost an afterthought) to a long list of problems and afflictions. But for us, balancing a focus on challenges with a process that elicits abilities, skills, and know-how at individual, relational, and sociocultural levels is profoundly important. Strengths are more than a cliché. Strengths represent a way forward.

RETHINKING STRENGTHS AND NEEDS

Helping organizations often organize their work around identifying strengths and needs to then develop a plan that draws on strengths to address needs. While this has a nice flow and is a time-honored tradition, we'd like to raise some concerns about this approach. When we begin with strengths in the abstract (Joanne is a good hockey player, John is a good cook), we can end up generating a list of strengths that may feel empty and hollow (e.g., Joanne is a good hockey player, but so what? What has that got to do with the problems that brought us here?). These sparse descriptions of strengths can contribute to a sense that strengths discovery is simply happy talk that romanticizes families and doesn't deal with the tough realities of life. We believe strengths-based work is too important to let it fall into these stereotypes. Similarly, compiling an extensive list of needs to be addressed can be overwhelming and demoralizing for everyone. It can sap energy and obscure hope, provoking a defensiveness that creates reluctance to even continue talking. "Needs" is a very slippery concept. Identification of needs can easily slide from personal needs to professional desires. "You need to stop drinking" may be as much a professional instruction as a person's need.

As an alternative, we suggest beginning by eliciting a vision that provides an agreed-upon focus for helping work. With such a vision in place, we can then recast needs as obstacles to that vision and strengths as supports for that vision. This way of discussing strengths has the potential to become much more relevant (e.g., In the past, Joanne has had trouble transitioning into new schools. In that context, her skill as a hockey player may help her make friends, feel more connected at school, and ease her transition.). Similarly, placing needs in the context of obstacles has the potential to help us move from collecting an exhaustive list of every need that could be addressed to a refined list of the most relevant obstacles that stand in the way of preferred directions in life. The rest of this chapter recasts problems and strengths as obstacles to and supports for desired lives. We hope to provide a context that will lead to more effective conversations about problems and richer descriptions of strengths.

CONVERSATIONS ABOUT PROBLEMS AS OBSTACLES SEPARATE FROM PEOPLE

In the process of "walking and talking" with people, our conversations are an important part of our work. However, the way we think about problems and people influences how we talk with them. The helping professions have traditionally thought about people as *having* a problem (he has Attention Deficit Disorder, she has Obsessive-Compulsive Disorder) or *being* a problem (she's a Borderline, he's an Alcoholic). When people's identities are fused with the problems in their lives, our work can get bogged down by despair or defensiveness. We are interested in finding ways to talk about problems that minimize blame and shame. This is not because we want to have "nice" conversations but because we want to have more effective conversations. One useful way of doing this is through the use of externalizing conversations, originally developed by Michael White and David Epston (1990) and subsequently refined by many other authors in the narrative therapy community (Freedman & Combs, 1996; Freeman, Epston, & Lobovits, 1997; Madsen 2007a; Monk, Winslade, Crocket, & Epston, 1997; Morgan, 2000; Russell & Carey, 2004; White, 2007; Zimmerman & Dickerson, 1996; to name a few). While these questions were originally developed in a therapy context, they have been expanded into a number of outreach and community settings. As described in Chapter 3, externalizing conversations offer a powerful way to help people address obstacles and develop proactive coping strategies. They are an attempt to separate problems from people in order for people to experience a sense of self outside the influence of a particular problem. This can be particularly useful in our work. When people experience themselves as *being in a relationship with* a problem rather than *having* or *being* a problem, they often experience a sense of relief and an increased ability to do something about the problem. Externalizing creates a space between people and problems that enables them to draw on previously obscured abilities, skills, and know-how to revise their relationship with the problem.

We want to emphasize that externalizing is much more than just a technique or intervention to be used with people. It represents a different approach to thinking about problems and the people affected by them. In this way, externalizing is perhaps most useful as a way to assist helpers in developing a different way of thinking about problems. The development of these habits of thought can have powerful effects on helping relationships. Thinking about obstacles to preferred directions in life as problems separate from people is likely to make a big difference in our work even if we don't engage in "official" externalizing conversations. Simply thinking in an externalizing fashion radically shifts how workers are positioned in helping relationships. At the same time, externalizing can be very useful in conversations between workers and people about problems in their lives. We hope to highlight this in a number of ways.

Beginning Externalizing Conversations

One way to begin externalizing conversations is to switch adjectives that people use into nouns. Here's a brief example of that process:

Father: I've had it up to here. I am so frustrated with my son.

Worker: What's happening that gets you so frustrated?

Father: Oh, he's doing A, B, and C.

Worker: And when he does A, B, and C, and that brings this Frustration in on you, what do you find yourself worrying about?[1]

Father: Oh, I worry about X, Y, and Z. My head is just filled with thoughts about them.

Worker: And when these Worrying Thoughts come into your head, how do you notice it? What's that like for you to have these Worries filling up your head?

Father: It sucks.

Worker: Yeah, how so? What's it like for you living with these Worrying Thoughts? Is that phrase, Worrying Thoughts, a good description for it?

From here the ground is set for a conversation about Worrying Thoughts as an entity separate from the person involved. In this process, it is important to draw on their language and make sure that the name for a problem is close to their own experience and fits for them.

We can also introduce externalizing conversations by contextualizing them. For example, we might say,

> At times people have found it helpful to think about problems like the one you're describing as separate things that can be personified in order to talk about them differently. So, for example, if the Worrying Thoughts were these outside things that crowd into your head and make life difficult as you've described, would that way of thinking about this situation make a difference for you? Sometimes people have found this way of talking about a problem to be really helpful. Would you like to try that and see if it works for you?

[handwritten margin note: Problems as seperate from individual.]

And some workers have found it useful to introduce externalizing conversations with stories from their own lives. Here's an example from Marianne, quoted in the last chapter, talking about her own experience trying to connect with gang-involved youth.

> I meet with a lot of youth who have been described as "having an anger management problem" or "being violent," when maybe what they did was protest or confront mistreatment by authorities in their lives. Externalizing helps shift the problem from the person to the oppressive context they live in. But, it can initially come across as very weird, so I've found it helpful to introduce it by talking about my own relationship with this thing that gets called "Violence." I'll tell them that from age 5, I was called violent. I had a violent jacket. People saw me and said, "She's violent." I started to believe I was violent and that violence was me. I was the poster child for violence. And I'll say to them, it wasn't until my 30s that I ran into someone who said, "Well, is it possible that you're influenced by violence and is there a name you would like to give it?" And that was a pretty wild idea and I said, "Yeah, it's like the Rhino." And I start talking about the Rhino. I don't call it rage or anger, but the Rhino. And the Rhino still tries to talk to me when I'm scared or feeling inadequate or minimized in some way. And the Rhino will say, "You know what you need to do? You need to correct the imbalance of power here and I can help you access intimidation and together we're really good at that." And this might seem kind of crazy, but the ability to talk to this part of me has been really helpful. I know its influence better than anybody. And when I lay it out like that,

it makes sense to people and they can then step into an externalizing conversation more easily.

*And when you introduce externalizing by talking about your own life, what's
your hope or intention in doing that?*

> Partly to equal out the playing field a little bit, to let this person
> know that helpers are human, too, and we're also dealing with
> things and that can ease the hierarchy of power. It leaves people
> with a sense of talking to a human being rather than someone
> who has already figured it all out. I don't ever want a person to
> be in a position of feeling "less than" me. I think they've had
> enough of that in life, so I do what I can and I think disclosure
> is a part of it. At the same time, I want to be really clear that this is
> not about my story. I'm disclosing stuff about me to connect
> with people through similar experiences, but I'm very clear that
> they're at the center of this, not me. And I've bumped heads
> with a lot of professionals who've said, "What you're doing is
> not good." Well, it's not good for them. They may like that
> position of power, but I don't.

We think Marianne raises some important and potentially provocative
issues here. Her introduction of externalizing through her own experience brings it down to a concrete level and makes it more real for
people. Her attention to how she positions herself with people and her
commitment to try to interact in ways that are not inadvertently disempowering have contributed to the perception on the street that she is
someone who "gets it and can be trusted." At the same time, this way
of interacting with people served may stretch the bounds of what has
traditionally been considered "appropriate" in helping practice and does
carry with it some important considerations that we take up more in the
next chapter.

Examples of Externalizing Conversations

One of the wonderful things about externalizing is the opportunities it
provides to creatively engage people with language that is accessible and
personally meaningful. We highlight some examples of this in conversations around problems, beliefs, interactional patterns, and broader dilemmas and situations.

Alex is an 8-year-old girl struggling with anxiety. She feels very
ashamed of the presence of anxiety in her life and doesn't want to talk

about it. Janice, an outreach worker, met with Alex and her mother, Mary. Mary had previously described her daughter's grand hopes for her upcoming summer break and her own worry that anxiety would subvert her daughter's plans. Mary also cautioned the worker Janice that the mere mention of anxiety would bring any conversation with Alex to an abrupt halt. After spending some time getting to know Alex and her mother and asking about their respective hopes for Alex's upcoming summer, Janice asked if there was anything that might get in the way of Alex's exciting plans. The question was greeted with an awkward silence, which was finally broken by the following exchange:

Janice: Alex, your mom told me that one of the things that might get in the way of your summer plans is this thing that other helpers have called "Anxiety." She also warned me that you weren't too keen on this label and might not want to talk to me at all about it. I'm more interested in hearing what you think about this than what others think. I'd like to ask you a couple questions about that and if you tell me to back off, I will. Would that be okay?

Alex: Okay, but I'm not anxious.

Janice: Okay, so this thing that other people call "Anxiety" but really might not be, how do you notice it in your life? When does it show up and what's it like when it's there?

Alex responded that sometimes she felt like she was caught in Saran Wrap and had no room to move. Janice asked if she could ask a bit more about that with the reminder that if Alex wanted her to back off, she would. This led into a long conversation about what this Saran Wrap Thingy was like for Alex, what effects it had on her, what she thought about those effects, and times when she had been able to stretch it out a bit and create more room to move in her life. Janice did this by pulling out some paper and engaging Alex to draw some pictures of herself caught in Saran Wrap, her reactions to that situation, and moments of her unwrapping herself a bit. At the end of the meeting, her mom commented on how openly Alex had talked about the Saran Wrap Thingy and Alex replied, "That's because we weren't talking about anything personal!" We would suggest that while this was an intensely personal conversation, it wasn't personalizing. The shift from professional language of "anxiety" to Alex's own language of "Saran Wrap" allowed her to enter into the conversation in a much more engaged fashion.

We can use externalizing conversations to discuss problematic beliefs. Emily is an employment counselor trying to help a young White lesbian woman, Terry, who had a very rough time when she came out to her parents and was subsequently fired from her job and doesn't see herself as deserving of much of anything. As Terry puts it, "I am so screwed up that no one would ever hire me. What's the use?" Rather than trying to convince Terry that this was not the case, Emily became very interested in this belief that Terry was "screwed up." She asked a number of questions about when this belief showed up in Terry's life (usually in the morning, especially if she didn't eat breakfast and returned to bed); what effects it had on her (desperation and hopelessness); when the belief was stronger in relation to Terry; when Terry felt stronger in relation to the belief; and which times she liked better. As Terry began to experience some distance between herself and this belief, and felt less captured by desperation and hopelessness, Emily wondered if there were times when Terry felt less like this was a belief that she was holding and more like a belief that was trying to hold her. Terry nodded enthusiastically and exclaimed, "Maybe it's not me who is screwed up. Maybe this Belief is screwed up." That led to a number of other questions on Emily's part such as:

- What might be screwed up about this Belief?
- You had mentioned having a hard time after coming out to your parents as gay. Do you think this Screwed Up Belief might get any support from the broader culture we live in?[2]
- What screwed up plans might this Belief have for your life?
- What tricks and tactics does it use to try to get you to buy into those plans?
- Do you think those tricks and tactics are fair, or screwed up?
- How did you come to take a stand against the screwed up ideas of this Belief?
- How are you continuing to make your own plans for your life, and what might be some next steps in those plans?

Externalizing questions [handwritten margin note]

We've listed out a set of questions that Emily asked. It's important to note these were not a series of rapid-fire questions, but questions that emerged in the conversation based on Terry's responses. While we may have some questions in mind as we start off this process, it is very important to keep it conversational and responsive to the person with whom we are talking. Emily later commented that at times she was tempted to hurry things along and just point out to Terry that this belief was indeed screwed up and that she should just let go of it, but as Emily put it, "Sometimes the quickest way to do things is not the quickest way." This is a good reminder for all of us. In the press of work, we can sometimes rush through things to get them done. We benefit from slowing down and staying present with people in order to ensure that the process is meaningful to them and not just something we have "checked off" and completed. Again, we come back to a focus on the process of these conversations rather than simply a product or outcome from them.

We can use externalizing conversations to address problematic interactions. These could be interactions between a couple, a caregiver and child, a helper and person served, or other permutations. Any time people interact over time, they often fall into repetitive patterns that can take on a life of their own and pull people into them.[3] We can think of these patterns as a series of mutual invitations (e.g., Person A's behavior invites Person B's response and Person B's response invites Person A's counterresponse). As these patterns take on a life of their own, we can shift from thinking about the "people doing the pattern" to the "pattern doing the people." In that context, we can externalize the pattern and examine its influence on the people involved as well as their efforts to get out from under the effects of those patterns, as in the following example.

Emil is a 70-year-old African-American man living on the south side of Chicago. He struggles with diabetes, complicated by a long relationship with alcohol in his life. When he drinks, his diabetes becomes unmanageable. Emil doesn't believe his drinking is a problem. His wife, Martha, on the other hand, worries enough for both of them. Emil responds to her concerns by minimizing the seriousness of his medical situation. They are caught in an over-responsible/under-responsible pattern in which the more she worries, the less concerned he appears, and the less he worries, the more her concerns escalate. The pattern between them is captured in Figure 6.1.

A primary care provider traces out this dance with them and they both agree that the pattern has negative effects on each of them as well as on their relationship. As Emil puts it, "I feel we can never relax. She's always monitoring me and I'm always waiting for the ax to fall." Martha quickly responds, "Yeah, but you don't know how much I hold my

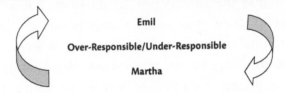

FIGURE 6.1   EXTERNALIZING AN OVER-RESPONSIBLE/
               UNDER-RESPONSIBLE PATTERN

tongue because everything I say gets immediately discounted. If I raise my concerns, I worry he'll just eat and drink more to prove he's his own man and if I don't raise my concerns, I worry I'm helping him kill himself. Neither choice works for me and my own health suffers as a result." As this interactional pattern was identified and examined with them, they both agreed that it had horrible effects on them and that they hated those effects. Stepping back from his reactivity to his wife's efforts, Emil became very concerned about the effects of this pattern on her health and decided to change his diet and cut back on his drinking as a way to support Martha's health. A year later, his hypertension is still high, but under better control than it has been in the past 5 years.

We can also use externalizing conversations to learn about dilemmas and problematic situations. Pedro is an undocumented Chicano man who works as a janitor in a large office building and lives in a homeless shelter. He describes repeated examples of feeling invisible as business people in the building walk across a floor he's just mopped, drop trash in a receptacle as he's attempting to change the trash bag, or ignore him as he's trying to get them to hold an elevator door. An outreach worker at the shelter asks him about the effects of Invisibility on him; the toll it takes on him; the broader economic, political, and sociocultural forces that support Invisibility; the ways in which Invisibility tries to "disappear" Pedro; as well as his efforts to remain a presence in his life despite Invisibility's best efforts. Pedro comments that the worker "gets it" and remarks, "This is the first time someone has really seen me since coming to this country." These conversations do not change broader systemic problems. For example, externalizing conversations alone will not end racism in Pedro's situation or homophobia in Terry's situation, but these conversations can go a long way to mitigating the devastating effects of these broader forces.

A MAP FOR EXTERNALIZING CONVERSATIONS ABOUT PROBLEMS

Externalizing conversations can sometimes feel unwieldy, leaving workers feeling lost and wanting to give up. Here is a simple map for these conversations that directs our questions to four areas: experience of the problem, effects of the problem, preferences about those effects, and responses to the problem. Figure 6.2 depicts the flow of these four areas of inquiry in which the questions begin at the top category and move clockwise.

We can begin by asking people about the ways in which they notice the presence of a particular problem and cast their description as a noun that can be seen as a separate entity. Then we can ask about how they have been affected by the problem's influence on their life and what they think about those effects. As we find ways in which those effects are not to their liking, we can then shift from questions about the influence of the problem on their life to questions about their influence on the life of the problem (i.e., ways in which they have continued to maintain a preferred life in the face of the problem). The remainder of this section outlines the purpose of each area of inquiry and highlights some questions that serve as examples.

Questions about people's experience of a problem seek to separate the problem from the person through externalizing language and develop a

---

FIGURE 6.2   **A MAP FOR EXTERNALIZING CONVERSATIONS**

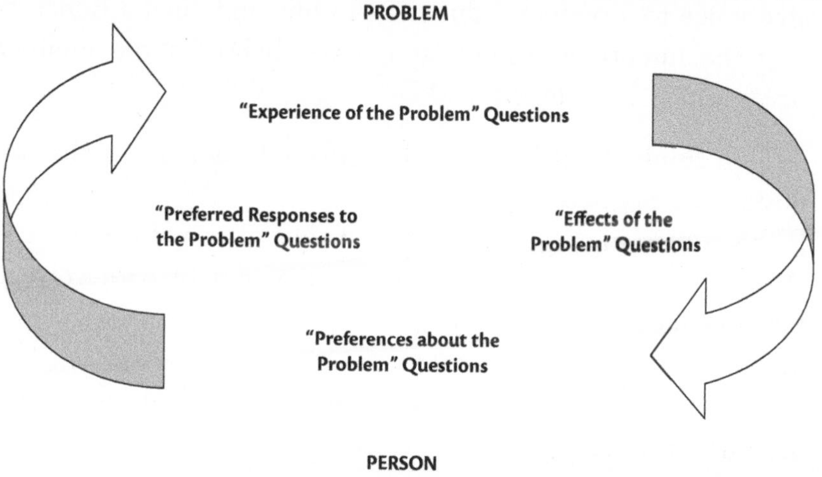

Adapted from W. C. Madsen (2007a). *Collaborative Therapy with Multi-Stressed Families, 2nd ed.*

rich understanding of that person's experience of his or her relationship with that problem. Generic examples (using XX to denote problems like Worry, Saran Wrap, that Screwed Up Belief, an Over-Responsible/Under-Responsible Pattern, Invisibility, Racism, Homophobia, etc.) include:

- When and where is XX most likely to come into your life?
- How can you tell when XX shows up?
- What's it like having XX in your life?

Questions about the effects of a problem seek to understand the toll a problem has taken on a person, on important others, and on relationships. Generic examples include: *Impact of problem on others*

- When XX comes into your life, how does that affect you?
- What has XX tried to get you to do that goes against your own better judgment?
- Has XX created problems for you in relationships? If so, in what ways?
- What does XX try to convince you about yourself? If XX were calling the shots in your life, where might it try to take you?
- If XX were to get even stronger over the next 6 months, how might that affect your life?

Questions about preferences invite people to reflect on the degree to which the effects of a problem fit with their own preferences in life.[4] These questions invite people to take a stand on the effects of a problem, give voice to a preferred direction in life, and elicit a richer explanation of the intentions, values, and hopes behind those preferences. Generic examples include: *How does the problem fit in with their life preferences.*

- As you think about how XX has affected your life, is that mostly positive or negative?
- Is this something you'd like more or less of in your life?
- Why is that? How do these effects fit or not fit with your hopes for your life?
- Where would you rather take your life?
- What do these preferences say about what you care for and value in your own life?

Preferred response questions seek to learn how people have responded to a problem and worked to maintain desired ways of living in the face of that problem's effects. These questions seek to elicit and elaborate on a story of their efforts to develop a different relationship with a problem (which may be to resist it, oppose it, overcome it, cope with it, contain or outgrow it, use it constructively, etc.), invite them to give meaning to this story, and examine future possibilities as that story unfolds. Generic examples include:

- You say that you don't like the effects of XX and that you would like to find a way to keep it in its place. Would it be okay if I ask you about some of the ways you do just that?
- Can you think of a time when you were able to keep XX in its place even if just a little bit?
- What did you do differently? How did you do that? Who and what helped you to do that?
- Was this something new or have there been other similar times? Would you tell me more about those times?
- What does it mean to you that you've been able to do this? What does it tell you about yourself?
- What capacities or abilities or know-how does it show? How did you develop those capacities? Who and what helped you in developing them?
- As you continue down this new path, how will that affect other parts of your life?

It is important to keep in mind that these sample questions are generic and need to be adapted to specific situations with language that is both close to people's daily experience and yet different enough to generate new experiences in the inquiry process. One initial reaction to these kinds of questions among helping professionals can be "These questions are weird. People don't talk like that in real life." That's right. These questions can be kind of awkward because they reflect a way of thinking about problems that is quite different from how many of us (especially in Western cultures that emphasize individualism and an internalized view of problems) have been socialized into thinking. The purpose of these questions is to invite people into a different way of thinking about problems, which hopefully contributes to a different experience of their relationship with those problems. The trick is to strike a balance between using language that is not off-putting and language that carries people outside their usual experience. This is an initial map for externalizing conversations. As workers develop more facility and comfort with

externalizing conversations, they can expand and draw on more complicated maps of externalizing conversations (Freedman & Combs, 1996;
Madsen, 2007a; Morgan, 2000; White, 2007).

Addressing the Broader Sociocultural Context in Externalizing

Obstacles occur at individual, relational, and sociocultural levels. These
are often intertwined and it is important to ask about the historical and
social context in which problems "live and grow." We saw the importance of sociocultural contexts in Terry's struggle with the Belief that
she is screwed up and in Pedro's struggle with Invisibility. In both of
these situations, the respective problems may receive significant support
in beliefs and attitudes in a broader culture that is struggling with accep-
tance of LGBT individuals and undocumented Latinos. Here is another
example of that kind of dynamic.

Mona is a poor White single mother who is distressed that her
8-year-old daughter Sonja is struggling in her life. Mona believes she is
to blame for her daughter's difficulties and feels doubly bad about her
daughter's troubles and her "obvious" culpability for them. In a conversation, a sympathetic outreach worker (who also has an 8-year-old
daughter) asks Mona whether she's gotten caught in blaming herself for
her daughter's difficulties. Mona nods and the worker asks her if she
knows other mothers who have had similar experiences. After an initial
"no," Mona reconsiders and proceeds through a laundry list of other
mothers she knows who at one time or another have blamed themselves
for their kids' struggles. Mona reflects on this and says, "You mean, this
is not just me?" Her outreach counselor, feeling the weight of the same
burden of "Mother Blame," nods and says, "Maybe not so much." As
they continue to talk about how Mona might not be the only mom
captured by Mother Blame, both Mona and her outreach worker are
very moved. Mona experiences this shift from "Mona as problematic"
to "Mona as captured by a problematic situation larger than her" as profoundly validating and confirming. She feels relieved and empowered
from the realization that this extends beyond her and is a problem she
shares with other women in her situation. In that context, she becomes
interested in connecting up with other single mothers and finding a way
to address the prevalence of Mother Blame in their lives.

Helping people to take a larger view of their lives can be profoundly empowering to them. We want to acknowledge that we live in a sociocultural context in which historically some people have come to matter less than others. We think this is a serious problem and one that interferes with efforts to help the people who have been most beaten down in our society. At the same time, we want to draw a clear distinction between asking questions that invite people to consider whether and how challenges in their life occur within and might be supported by a broader sociocultural context and trying to get them to arrive at a particular conclusion about their situation. The latter (pushing a particular agenda) is a misuse of helping power (since we as helpers are in a more privileged and less vulnerable position in relation to the people we serve, despite our subjective experience of the interaction). The former (asking questions about larger sociocultural considerations) represents an important expansion of helping practice and is a constructive use of helping power. The important issue here is not necessarily what conclusions are arrived at, but what questions and considerations are raised. In the spirit of Karl Tomm's distinction between corrective and facilitative questions in Chapter 2, we are focused here on opening space for different possibilities to emerge rather than trying to determine how people should live their lives.

CONVERSATIONS ABOUT STRENGTHS AS INTENTIONAL PRACTICES OF LIVING

While the helping field has typically focused more on problems and obstacles, we can also elicit strengths and supports in people's lives. We want to suggest the usefulness of a shift from viewing strengths as *characteristics* to viewing strengths as *practices* (i.e., things people do in their lives). The shift from viewing strengths as characteristics (something a person *is*) to viewing strengths as intentional practices (something a person *does* backed by intentions, values and beliefs, hopes and dreams, and commitments in life) can lead to more poignant conversations about strengths, and assist people in cultivating and further developing those strengths. We can begin these conversations by inquiring about either supports for preferred directions in life or exceptions to obstacles (i.e., times when people have been a bit more able to resist the pull of a particular problem). We take a look at this in action, highlight a map to guide conversations about strengths and supports, and offer several other examples of this process in different contexts and at different levels (individual, relational, and sociocultural, which of course are always intertwined).

Determination as a Counterweight to Despair

In Chapter 5, we discussed Margie, a Polish-American woman struggling with uncontrolled Diabetes, who was caught in a minimize/maximize pattern with her husband Walter about her medical condition. The conflict contributed to her belief that her hopes for retirement with travel to Italy (long a dream for both of them) had been stolen away and that she was condemned to a retirement of increased disability and eventual death. In this context, an outreach nurse Kristen learned about her efforts to go with her husband on outings to the North End, an Italian section of Boston, as an act of resistance to the distressing situation she felt life had in store for her. The last chapter examined this development as an emerging exception to a "No Control Stance." This section highlights some ways in which Kristen, the outreach nurse, built on this exception to identify strengths that could support Margie and Walter in pursuing their dream of a retirement life of travel.

Before getting into the details of how Kristen approached this, we want to say something about the broader assumptions that shaped her work. Much of Margie's time with Kristen had been focused on how bad and unfair things were for her. One of the things we want to emphasize in this consideration of strengths is that people's sense of self is continually changing. Whether we are talking about strengths or problems, if we consider them inherent personality characteristics, we lock ourselves into a fairly fixed and limiting conceptualization of life. If we think about identity as something that develops and continually evolves in a social context (*how* we are rather than *who* we are), we open up more possibilities and options for responding to life's challenges. Kristen was able to see Margie's complaints about her life situation in a social context. She believed that while Margie at times felt few to no options in life, this was not the whole story of her life. Kristen actively sought out exceptions to this dominant story. As Margie talked about her North End outings, Kristen viewed those outings as another description or story about her life. It is important for helpers to be able to hold multiple realities simultaneously. In this context, we can view Margie as both locked into a limiting view of possibilities in life and, at the same time, actively resisting that situation and seeking alternatives. What becomes important is what we choose to highlight. Kristen's choice was to acknowledge the power of a story of No Control Stance in Margie's life and highlight exceptions to that story.

In a conversation over the kitchen table, Margie mentioned outings to the North End. While this was a small thing that could be easily overlooked, Kristen picked up on it and asked Margie, "As you think about your commitment to keeping alive your Italy dreams by going to the North End, is there a word or phrase that for you captures that commitment? Like what is that about for you?" Margie immediately responded, "Determination. I'm determined not to let these dreams just die. I'm determined to keep them alive." Kristen responded, "You seem really clear in that statement. At times you've talked pretty pessimistically about your situation, and yet here you are talking with incredible clarity about Determination to keep your dreams alive. Can I ask you more about that?" With Margie's assent, they began to talk about some of the concrete ways that Margie had cajoled Walter into taking her to the North End. After some hilarious tales about Margie's creative efforts, Kristen asked her about her hopes and intentions in those efforts. Margie described her desire to make a better life for her husband and herself in the time they had left together. As she put it,

> My husband worked his whole life at some crappy job (please don't tell him I said that) so that we could retire and travel. Going to Italy has been our dream for many years. I don't know how much longer I'm going to be around with this diabetes and all, but I'd rather spend that time living rather than avoiding dying. So, I thought we could do the best we could with what was available and that was going out to dinner in a neighborhood we could pretend was Italy.

Kristen said she was very moved by what she had just heard and wondered what about that was important to Margie. Margie thought and responded,

> Listen, I know I'm going to get older and more disabled and die some day. I don't need some expert to tell me that. Isn't that kind of what life is? For me the question is how I spend my life between now and then. I mean, I guess there are some things I could do to manage my diabetes better, but I'm tired of my life simply being some illness. My life is bigger than that.

At this point, both were close to tears and Kristin commented on Margie's statement that her life was bigger than simply being some illness and asked if Margie had any ideas on how together they could help her stay bigger than Diabetes. Margie responded by saying, "I don't know. Do you have any ideas about things I could do to help me manage this Diabetes?" This was the first time Margie had asked any healthcare provider for help in managing her Diabetes rather than just sitting passively through a lecture about what she should be doing differently. Kristin saw Margie as struggling with a retirement problem rather than simply a medical problem. In that context, she was able to tailor her helping efforts around Diabetes in the service of something much more important to Margie. In continued kitchen table conversations, she helped Margie build on her "Determination to Live" in support of dreams of travel. They talked about ways in which Margie could alter her diet and lifestyle in order to live out her hopes for a trip with her husband. Currently, Margie is managing her medical condition (with periodic slips) and has taken one weeklong trip to Italy with another planned for next year. While these kitchen table conversations were very informal, they were also quite thoughtful and purposeful. The next section outlines a broad map to help us reconsider strengths as "intentional practices of living" and to have conversations that open possibilities for people to use these strengths to build lives they would prefer.

A Map for Conversations About Strengths

Kristen's conversations with Margie were grounded in a spirit of respect, connection, curiosity, and hope and that had a huge impact on the effectiveness of those conversations. At the same time, she had a broad map in her head to organize her questions in a way that helped her embody that spirit. We can identify three broad areas of inquiry in conversations about strengths and supports:

1. Identifying strengths as practices (e.g., things people do in their lives)
2. Eliciting possible intentions, values and beliefs, hopes and dreams, and commitments in life that might stand behind those practices
3. Developing a community that can support people in those intentional practices

We can begin these conversations by turning adjectives (e.g., I'm determined) into nouns (e.g., "Determination" as an externalized entity) and then further turning those nouns into active verb processes. Here are some sample generic questions to help us accomplish that:

- Can you tell me more about this Determination?
- If Determination was not a quality that you have, but something you do, how do you do that? For you, what are the practices of Determination?
- How did you develop those practices?
- Who and what contributed to the development of those practices?
- What makes that important to you?

Practices in life come and go. We all have way too many experiences of committing to a practice (e.g., I'm going to exercise regularly) that falls away. Here are some questions to help people sustain supportive practices (or strengths) by eliciting important intentions, values and beliefs, hopes and dreams, and commitments in life that stand behind them:

- When you were doing this Determination, what was your intention? What were you trying to accomplish? What was your hope in that?
- As you think about those intentions, what values and beliefs might sit behind them?
- When you think of those values, what hopes or dreams might they reflect?
- What might those hopes and dreams say about what you are committed to or what you stand for in your life?

The movement from practices (What are you doing?) to intentions (Why are you doing that? What are your intentions in doing that? What are you hoping to accomplish in doing that?) can be difficult and yet very important. Sometimes, questions about intentions can feel patently obvious. At the same time, they provide an important foundation for further questions about values and beliefs, hopes and dreams, and commitments in life. This progression of questions was developed by Michael White (2007) and helps us engage in very meaningful conversations about strengths in a short period of time. This particular progression (intentions > values and beliefs > hopes and dreams > commitments in life) is very deliberate. Each set of questions sets a stage for subsequent questions and encourages small steps that support people's ability to consider and respond to these questions. At the same time, this flow represents an overall guideline. They are principles to guide a conversation, not a recipe to be simply followed. Using these questions in a stepped progression without attention to the people's responses usually has problematic results. This is where the idea of "disciplined improvisation" originally described in Chapter 2 reenters. It is important to strike a balance between holding a disciplined map that guides our questioning process and an improvisational practice that accommodates unexpected responses.

From here, we can further embed the "practices" of strengths by developing a community of support for them. Here are some sample generic questions for that as pertains to Determination:

- As you think back across your life, who do you think might particularly appreciate your pursuit of Determination in the face of the fear and anxiety provoked by Diabetes?
- How have those people contributed to your development of Determination?
- If they could witness you putting Determination into practice, what do you think it would tell them about you?
- What's it like for you to be thinking and talking about them right now?
- Would you like to have their presence more in your life? If so, what could help you do that?

APPLICATIONS OF CONVERSATIONS ABOUT STRENGTHS

We can begin conversations about strengths by inquiring about supports for preferred directions in life or exceptions to obstacles to preferred directions in life. Here are several examples of eliciting, elaborating, and acknowledging supports at individual, relational, and sociocultural levels (knowing that they are all interconnected and this distinction is a bit of an artificial one).

Committed to the Practice of Self-Care—Building on Supports at an Individual Level

This example highlights a conversation with an individual about positive steps toward a preferred direction in life. Charlie is a punk rocker who has struggled with substance misuse for many years. Frankie is an outreach substance abuse counselor who has been influenced by narrative approaches to substance misuse (Butterworth, 2000; Crowe, 2006; Mankwong, 2004) and who works within a harm reduction program dedicated to helping people minimize the harmful effect of substances in life without demanding abstinence. Charlie does a lot of various drugs and has a strong commitment to a life of continued drug use that doesn't consume his life. Frankie, being quite cautious about the dangers of Drugs taking over Charlie's life, agrees to work with him to minimize harm with the proviso that if it seems their work is inadvertently supporting Drugs rather than Charlie, they will renegotiate. Being very influenced by Paul Butterworth's (2000) work on self-care, Frankie engages Charlie in a conversation about the ways in which he reduces the toll that Drugs take on his life. He frames this in terms of "self-care" and focuses his conversations on the ways in which Charlie draws on Self-Care to get to a life in which he is "happy, self-supportive, and responsible to others in his life" (a goal Charlie had articulated).

Frankie elicits the ways in which Charlie engages in the practice of Self-Care and gets detailed descriptions of those practices. He elicits Charlie's intentions ("I want to live a life of exploration."), values and beliefs ("We're on this planet for a purpose, let's find out what it is."), hopes and dreams ("We would live our life to our fullest and be conscious about how we're affecting others."), and commitments ("I want to be a person on this planet who is kind."). In this context, Frankie engages Charlie in a conversation about the ways in which Charlie's daily activities support or contradict those intentions, values and beliefs, hopes and dreams, and commitments and asks him about the person he'd most like to be. Charlie responds with crystal clarity, "I'm not going to stop getting high, but this planet is a delicate place and I don't want to mess that up. I've done some awful stuff to people when I'm high, which I didn't recognize at the time. That's screwed up and I feel really bad about that. I'm going to ask (Charlie mentions three friends) to help me hold true to the ways I want to be in the world and check in with them on a regular basis." These are notable ambitions and ones that can easily get lost in everyday life. Frankie helped Charlie build on this expressed commitment and go further to actually develop a way to regularly check in with these three friends about their sense of how he was doing in his life.

Stepping Off the Merry-Go-Round—Building on Supports at a Relational Level

This example comes out of an exception to a problematic interactional pattern in a family. Ayisha is a 13-year-old African-American youth in an inner city neighborhood who is caught up in significant struggles with her mother and grandmother with whom she lives. They have all become caught in a repetitive pattern in which Ayisha misbehaves (drinking, smoking pot, shoplifting, etc.) and her mother and grandmother respond by labeling her as "bad, stupid, and unmotivated." She in turn responds to their accusations by taking a stance of "I don't care." The more her mother and grandmother come down on her, the more disinterested she becomes, which in turn leads to more outrage and worry on her mother's and grandmother's part. In talking with the family, an outreach worker traces out the pattern and asks them what they think about the effects of this pattern on their family. While they have different ideas about what causes this pattern and who should be blamed for it, they all agree that it has extremely negative effects on their relationships and that they don't like it. They describe it as "being on a Merry-Go-Round that never stops."

Their outreach worker replies, "Given that you don't like the effect of the Merry-Go-Round on each of you and your family, are there times when you've been able to step off that Merry-Go-Round and do something different?" They initially had difficulty identifying such a time, but with persistent patience and encouragement from their outreach worker, they described a time when Ayisha and an older cousin asked to go to a convenience store (which was next to a local liquor store) to get an ice cream. They were initially quite hesitant to give permission, fearing the young folks would actually go to get alcohol, but laid out their concerns and agreed to pay for the ice cream with a promise the kids wouldn't get alcohol. When subsequently asked about it,

Ayisha said, "I get that they have a hard time trusting me and I guess that makes some sense. I liked that they were willing to take a chance and I didn't want to blow that." Her mother said, "My mom was pretty suspicious, but I wanted to give Ayisha a vote of confidence. I figured if I said no, she'd be likely to go get some alcohol later and if I laid out why I was concerned, it might take us somewhere different." In juxtaposing this new interaction with the old "Merry-Go-Round" interaction, the outreach worker asked what phrase they might use to describe this interaction and they said, "The Trust-Go-Round. We trust her, she rewards our trust, and we trust her more."

The worker traced out the interaction in detail (who said what, how others responded in turn, responses to responses, etc.) and asked what was important to them about a "Trust-Go-Round" interaction. She asked Ayisha, her mother, and her grandmother about the respective intentions behind the steps they took, what values might stand behind those intentions, and what hopes and dreams for their family might be reflected in those values. Following that, the outreach worker asked them who might not be surprised to hear about the development of the Trust-Go-Round. Ayisha's mom said that her father, who had passed away a year ago and was very close to both Mother and Ayisha, would be very encouraged to hear about the Trust-Go-Round and she described how holding his confidence in Ayisha helped her to have faith in her daughter. Ayisha, in turn, spoke about the ways in which evoking the presence of her grandfather warmed her heart and left her feeling like she didn't want to disappoint either him or her mother.

Rolling It Off Your Back—Building on Supports at a Sociocultural Level

We can also draw on supports that grow out of enduring cultural values. An example of this comes from the story of Frieda, an African-American woman who described numerous examples of being summoned to school meetings about her children who were struggling in a predominantly White school. She reflected on her experience of walking into the school and feeling like other parents and school personnel were treating her in a very unwelcoming fashion. When asked if this bothered her, she replied, "No, it just rolls off my back. I got bigger fish to fry when I'm going to those meetings." Her Latina worker, who also had multiple experiences of racial micro-aggressions in her own life, asked Frieda how she rolls things off her back. Notice the difference between "things rolling off your back" and "rolling things off your back." If Frieda experiences herself as rolling things off her back, she becomes a more active participant in her life. It highlights her sense of agency and influence over parts of her life and opens space to examine the practices of rolling things off her back and how she developed that ability.

Framing this as an intentional practice enhances the possibility that Frieda can further cultivate this capacity and bring it into other areas of her life. Following up on her initial question, the worker commented to Frieda, "You know, sometimes things roll off my back, but other times they stick and really get under my skin. How are you able to roll it off your back?" She continued with other questions like "How do you do that? What goes into doing that? What helps you do that?" In this context, Frieda talked about how she stands on the shoulders of her mother and how her mother stood on the shoulders of her mother and how she hopes her children will be able to stand on her shoulders. She connected this to a deep family and cultural value of acknowledging the legacy of previous generations and carrying that legacy forward for future generations. She remarked that being grounded in that legacy helped her focus and not to get sidetracked by how she was received at the school. As she put it: "I said, I've got bigger fish to fry. I'm there to get my kids a fair break and I have to keep my back strong and uncluttered so my shoulders are available to them." In this way, tapping into broader cultural values supports her in being the kind of presence she wants to be for her children.

New Conversations About Problems and Strengths

We have examined some new ways of talking with people about the obstacles and supports in their lives. We want to emphasize again that these conversations are not simply techniques. The process of viewing people as separate from and more than the problems in their lives enhances connection and thereby can contribute to the development of very different helping relationships. Externalizing goes a long way toward minimizing the shame and blame associated with problems while also keeping a focus on people's responsibility to address those problems. Similarly, we can also think about strengths in an externalizing fashion and then move to seeing them as practices in living (things people are doing) rather than simply as personality characteristics. This shift in thinking leads to a richer consideration of strengths and can help people further cultivate them. Simply thinking about problems and strengths in these ways can be very useful.

At the same time, these actual conversations may be very helpful in people's lives. While they are based on a quite different way of thinking about problems and strengths and may feel initially awkward for helpers new to them, we'd encourage you to try them sometime and see how it goes. We've offered a simple map for *separating* people from obstacles that takes us through a conversation about how people notice or experience a particular problem, to the effects that problem has on them, to what they think about those effects and whether it suits them or not, and, if they don't like those effects, how they might prefer to respond to the problem and shift their relationship with it. These conversations can become very helpful in their lives. Similarly, we have examined a simple map for *connecting* people to supports in their lives by talking about strengths as practices, and then engaging people in conversations about particular intentions, values and beliefs, hopes and dreams, and commitments in life that might stand behind those practices as well as identifying important others who might stand in support of them. We hope that the outlines for these conversations help to push your work forward and create opportunities to engage in some very different conversations about both problems and strengths.

◾ NOTES

1. As we highlighted in Chapter 3, when we are talking about a particular problem in an externalizing fashion, we will capitalize it.
2. Placing problems in their broader sociocultural context and raising questions about ways in which take-for-granted assumptions in that broader context might support a problem is important and can be very helpful in this work. We note this now and take it up in more detail later in this chapter.
3. Madsen (2007a) offers a more extensive description of these kinds of sequences or patterns in Chapter 2 of his book. Much of that work was based on Karl Tomm's (1991) development of an alternative to DSM based on a taxonomy of interactional patterns (PIPs—problematic interactional patterns—and HIPs—healing interactional patterns) rather than a taxonomy of people.
4. Within the narrative literature, preference questions have been discussed in the context of "statement of position maps," in which people are asked to evaluate the effects of a problem and then justify their evaluation (White, 2007). We refer to them here as preference questions.

CHAPTER 7

Dilemmas in Home and Community Services

So far, we've developed ideas about an overall approach to helping and discussed practical ways to engage people in a helping relationship. We've talked about ways to develop a shared vision and talk differently about problems and strengths. We've emphasized the importance of inquiry as a way to guide helping efforts, moving from advising people on how to live their lives to asking questions that help them reflect on their own hopes and preferences in life, which enables them to then identify obstacles and supports in order to develop a concrete plan for drawing on those supports to address the obstacles that stand in the way of their getting to the vision they've described. We've called this process "walking and talking," referring to a combination of concrete assistance and thoughtful conversations with a focus on how people experience their lives and sense of self with an intention to walk with them as they step into life stories that open up more possibilities. This walking and talking is particularly applicable in outreach settings where workers have more flexibility in their time and are more involved in the immediacy of people's lives. This chapter examines some of the ways in which frontline workers can provide concrete services and engage in advocacy issues with people. We examine the terrain of home and community work and how it is different from office-based work. We particularly focus on how that different terrain calls into question traditional notions about professional boundaries and examine some of the boundary dilemmas that outreach workers encounter and how they respond to them.

We also examine advocacy efforts with a focus on ways to advocate *with* people rather than becoming the spokesperson for their interests. We take a look at some of the dilemmas faced by frontline helpers when advocating for people in a helping system in which the helpers themselves often have little influence and power. And we explore innovative ways to better help people advocate for themselves.

Concrete Help, Boundaries, and the Terrain of Home and Community Work

At times when people are overwhelmed by life's demands, concretely helping out with those challenges while also engaging in thoughtful conversation can be incredibly useful. The story from Chapter 1 of Amanda, a woman who was struggling in many ways, provides an example of this. Amanda's outreach worker Beth believed in her ability to rebuild a productive life and helped her begin community college. When Amanda initially said she'd never be able to do it, Beth responded with "Sure you can, I'll go with you to register and we'll talk about it on the way." Beth later described her thinking.

> We have the ability in our job to accompany people on their journeys. A scary journey can be not so scary if you have someone walking with you. We can help start the process when people have no sense of how to begin and they then pick up and build on it. It's empowering to have someone say, "We can do this. It might be a little scary, but we'll get through it." Amanda later told me that at the time she borrowed my belief in her to believe in herself. I thought that was really powerful.

In another situation, a CPS worker described going out to a home to meet with a mother, who had four young children, was involved with CPS because of issues of neglect, was struggling with depression, and had recently endured major surgery. When the worker came in, the mother was lying on the couch and there was a large collection of dirty dishes in the sink. The mother was exhausted and having a hard time recovering from surgery. With the mother's permission, the worker began washing the dishes as she talked with the mother about her recovery and how she might get some assistance from friends and neighbors for herself and her children during this time. The mother had been very hesitant to reach out to others, but when she saw the worker's willingness to chip in without seeming overly burdened by it, she became more open to turning to others in her community for help and they brainstormed a concrete plan for that to occur.

In both these situations, workers jumped in to provide concrete assistance in that moment. Helping people with immediate demands in their lives builds connection and establishes our relevance to them in the very real challenges of the day. It can also be a validating experience for people who too often feel blamed and shamed by helping systems. The willingness to pitch in and help out gives people a sense that "I'm not alone and maybe we can do this together." Helping becomes something concrete and understandable. The process of working in this way requires some rethinking of how our field has historically thought about "professional boundaries" in helping efforts. For example, some readers might wonder about a helping professional doing dishes while a "client" lies on the couch watching her. However, the worker in this instance described the conversation that unfolded as one of the best ones they'd had about better addressing neglect issues in the family and reaching out to others for help. She attributed the success of the conversation directly to her jumping in to help while the mother was in the midst of a painful and exhausting recovery from surgery. Let's take a look at how professional boundaries and the relationships we develop with people are different in home and community work and highlight particular dilemmas that frontline workers encounter and how they respond.

The Terrain of Home and Community Work

Working with people in home and community settings is quite a bit different from office-based work. When we meet with people in our office, there is a set of unspoken rules and agreements that we can count on. In home and community work, the rules are quite different and sometimes hard to understand. Here are two examples from an experienced home-based worker.

> When I was back in school, I learned that if a "patient" offered you a cup of coffee and you accepted, then treatment was over. These days, when I'm going out to people's homes, it's real clear to me that if a person offers you a cup of coffee and you decline, the work is over.
>
> When I did clinic work, I never had anyone show up in my office in their underwear. People generally get dressed before they get on a bus to go to an appointment. But, in seeing people

in their homes, there have been times when I've knocked on the door and have been greeted by someone in their "next to nothings."

The two stories playfully highlight how the terrain of home and community work tends to be more complicated. While many of the old rules may not apply so well, we still need guidelines and a clear place to stand in unanticipated situations. In fact, the relative lack of external structure and the absence of hard and fast rules confirm the importance of a principle-based approach to boundaries. Another story from a mother describing the most helpful interaction she ever had with a professional drives this home.

> My CPS worker left a meeting at my house and came running back and said, "I have a bureaucratic meeting downtown and snagged my nylons on my car door resulting in a horrible run. Do you have a pair of pantyhose I could borrow?" I didn't know if she was serious or if it was some kind of trick to connect with me, but if it was the latter, I have to say it was brilliant. It was the most powerful thing any professional has ever said to me. It equalized things between us and left me feeling like I had something to contribute (even though I couldn't help her out with the pantyhose). It was a turning point in our relationship and the most helpful interaction I've ever had with a professional.

While we do not encourage this encounter as some promising new engagement tactic, the fact that this mother considers this exchange the most helpful interaction she ever had with a professional is hard to ignore. As helping professionals, we are often encouraged to take up a dispassionate posture in the name of objectivity and good boundaries. An outreach worker in Mexico describes this stance as "stone face." She says, "When meeting with people, I show many different faces—the face of a caring neighbor, an aunt, or a loving grandmother, but I try to never show a stone face." When Bill related this story to a shelter worker back home, she responded, "That's not a stone face, it's a slap in the face for the people we serve." Showing our own humanity is not just good manners; it builds connection and a foundation for effective work. It also has powerful effects on the people we serve. When helpers step out from behind a professional persona and into a more shared relationship, people experience themselves differently. It encourages the development of more constructive life stories. We have consistently called for a deliberate shift in the way we relate to people from being the established expert to being an appreciative ally. Good things are more likely to happen when people move away from a "less than" experience to one where they feel supported. People feel supported when helpers relate to them in a personal way, believe in the possibility of a better life for them, and offer opportunities to actively make a contribution to a shared relationship. Interestingly, these three elements (supportive relationships, high expectations with a belief that people can meet them, and having opportunities to contribute) are factors that have been consistently found to contribute to resilience (Benard, 2004; 2006).

Boundary Dilemmas in Home and Community Work

An advocate in a drop-in center for women living on the street that we'll call "Safe Space" captures this reconsideration of boundaries:

> Most agencies have boundary lines. I think we have boundary ropes that we can tighten or loosen as we need depending on the individual we're dealing with and the relationship we have with them.

A more flexible definition of boundaries creates opportunities but also poses challenges and dilemmas. Let's see some of the ways frontline helpers have encountered and responded to such challenges. We'll begin with a story from a CPS worker that captures some of the ways a deeper connection can feel overwhelming.

> Being deeply connected to people is very meaningful, but the downside for me is now I know their story and it has a heavier burden on my heart to actually know them. Instead of us going in there and telling them what to do, we're engaging and listening, and when you do that, you feel their pain and sometimes that can be heartbreaking.

This helping worker emphatically stated that while it can be hard, she believes that feeling connected helps her do better work. Given the choice of showing her heart and carrying a heavier burden or hiding her heart and risk losing it, she has chosen the former. Susan, another Safe Space advocate, adds,

> I think being connected to people is an antidote to burnout because when a relationship is real and there's mutuality around it, it's more satisfying for both the worker and the person you're

in a relationship with. I leave at the end of the day feeling like I love my work because I love the people I work with and I feel like they love me and I'm not kidding. I feel like there is true love here in a way that is sustaining.

A common dilemma described by helpers who rely less on fixed rules to clarify boundaries is the need to be really clear about when you do and don't feel comfortable. Ashley, also from Safe Space, relates,

> Sometimes it's hard for me because I see our women every-where—on the train, riding my bike around town, and just moving through my life. I see them and because of how we approach the work, I stop and chat with them and sometimes that chatting gets in the way of getting my errands done. While I want to be kind and I am very interested in them, sometimes I have to be like, "Gotta go, see you tomorrow."

She describes this as requiring her to "be 'on' which can be hard, but probably good for me."

An outreach worker, in a different context, explains that he asks a lot of questions but always gives people the option to "pass." He tells people they can ask him questions, too. But he retains the all-important "pass" option as well. He relates a particular story about a man who was once heavily into the music and the culture of the Grateful Dead and who was using drugs and alcohol pretty heavily. The man asked the helper if he had any experience with drugs in his own life. The helper responded, "Well, I came of age in San Francisco in the early 70s, so it'd be kind of hard not to." He explained that response in the following way.

> I saw his question as asking me if I could connect with his experience and I wanted to respond in a way that conveyed that maybe I could. In that instance, that was the end of it. If he had pressed me for details, I probably would have passed. I have to sort out why he might ask me that question and how I can respond in ways that feel okay to me. Telling him, "That's an inappropriate question" or saying, "I'm wondering why you might ask that question?" is really off-putting. If I see this as an attempt to see whether we can connect, it's an opportunity to move forward. If I see this as an attempt to "bust" me, I can fall into dodging his question and that's not helpful. People usually ask questions like that because they just want to know who you

are and if you can possibly understand their life. Until it's proven otherwise, I'm going to assume people have positive intentions.

Helping workers tell us that when we are overly fearful of messy interactions, we miss opportunities for the connection that can happen when we step into a more open stance. Susan, from Safe Space, captures this idea.

> I would so much rather work in a place where I was being thoughtful about decisions I need to make related to this particular person than have a blanket way of how I'm going to treat everybody I work with. I don't think there is anything more powerful than being curious about other people's experience, making room for them to share and to feel truly listened to and connected with. In my work, I try to create every opportunity I can to be curious, to be a listener, to be a connector, to be a responder to what people are sharing with me in a way that lets them know it matters to me.

Another dilemma involves pouring heart and soul into a strong helping connection and then needing to take steps (e.g., involuntary hospitalizations) that might threaten that relationship. A shelter worker for people living on the street puts it this way.

> I bust my butt to build relationships with the folks I serve and then someone goes off their medication and is standing in traffic in front of our place and refusing to get out of the street. So, I go and gently pull them off of the street and then I have this dilemma. I really care about them, but have to make sure they're safe, and so maybe I should see about getting them hospitalized. I worry that if I do take steps to insure their safety, it'll threaten our relationship and if I don't take steps to insure their safety, it'll threaten their existence.

That's a tough dilemma. How do you deal with that?

> I try to lay it out for them. I say, "Here's the deal. You've had a lot of people in your life taking control away from you and I don't want to do that. You've also had a lot of people who just disappeared when you were in the midst of a hard time and I don't want to do that either. So, I feel like we're in a bind here. If I act, it could feel like I'm yet another person taking control away from you and I don't want to do that. If I don't act, it

could feel like I'm yet another person who has left you unprotected in your life and you've told me you are tired of that. So, this presents quite a dilemma for us. What do you think we might do together here?" Ultimately, I'm going to make the decision but bringing them into the process helps.

This worker said that simply laying out dilemmas encourages people to step into participating in a possible resolution and also helps to keep the relationship on track. The goal is not necessarily to completely resolve tension, but to name it and acknowledge its effects.

Finally, a pernicious and disheartening situation that occurs all too often in helping work involves amazing engagement efforts that are not only unappreciated by members of the larger helping system, but frequently criticized or even undermined. Here are two such stories.

An outreach worker goes to visit Dave, a father involved with Child Protective Services. She knocks on the door and a voice (sounding remarkably like Dave) asks, "Who's there?" She replies, "This is Miranda and I have an appointment with Dave today." In a response eerily reminiscent of the old Cheech and Chong comedy sketch, she hears, "Dave's not here." She responds, "Okay, would you tell him I'll come back this afternoon before my meeting with Child Protective Services?"

Another outreach worker knocks on an apartment door and is greeted by a woman holding a joint and looking quite surprised. The worker says, "Oh, I see I've caught you at a bad time. Why don't I come back in a half-hour?"

Both workers were very clear that they would need to have serious discussions with these two people about these interactions and they both felt like initiating those discussions in that moment would not go anywhere. At the same time, both of these workers faced significant criticism for "colluding" with people served. They were told, "You need to confront them and let them know that behavior is not okay." When asked about that criticism, one of them said,

You think they don't know that behavior was not okay? They were embarrassed and trying to cover. I don't want to back people into corners in trying to help them change. I always want to give them opportunities to save face and think about how I can help them be the best person they can in that moment. I'm not about catching them messing up, I'm about helping them move forward.

When asked what helps her remember that and not get caught by the criticism, she responded,

> I need to keep my focus on the long game. If I can bite my tongue in the moment and use our relationship as a foundation for a more constructive conversation down the line, that seems much more effective. I know from experience that approach works better and it's important to move at the pace I know works best.

As you think back over the various dilemmas described here, what crosscutting themes do you notice? Perhaps some core principles could be best summed up in the following bumper sticker: "Be real, be clear, and know your own limits." Experience tells us that genuineness is helpful. Clarity about what people can and can't expect from helpers makes for a much better relationship. And that requires clarity on the part of helping workers about their own comfort zone.

The Contribution of Family Partners to Collaborative Helping

As we move into examining the role of advocacy efforts and dilemmas that emerge, we need to first introduce the contributions of family partners in this work and see what we can learn from some of their experiences. The term *family partner* or *parent partner* comes out of wraparound work where organizations hire parents with children who have struggled with severe emotional distress to take on a supportive role with families. Often paired with a professionally trained care coordinator, they have been invaluable in both engaging families and helping agencies rethink taken-for-granted ideas and ways of working. Ellen Walnum (2007), a Norwegian woman who has worked in a context focused on helping families where a parent rather than a child has had "mental health difficulties," refers to this role as an "experience consultant." While her context is somewhat different, we think her contribution to our thinking about this role is profoundly helpful. In her work, she shares her life experiences with parents with psychiatric difficulties and their children, and with other professionals. The purpose in these efforts is to connect with and support people seeking help and to assist other helpers develop a richer understanding of what it might be like to go through such situations in life.

Programs that have successfully incorporated family partners or experience consultants have come to realize the significant contribution they can make in bringing experiential knowledge as well as professional knowledge to the table and legitimizing both kinds of knowledge. In this way, programs can benefit from both learned experience (things helpers learn in school and training) and lived experience (things people have learned in the course of living their lives). While both types of knowledge are important, the latter is often sidelined with an emphasis on the former. However, lived experience has much to contribute to our knowledge base. As Paulo Freire (1981) put it, "You learn to swim in the water, not in the library."

While the incorporation of family partners into wraparound programs may have been originally developed to help families, this development also has had significant effects on community agencies. Family partners have a unique position within the helping system. They have been in a position of being helped and now are a helping professional. Their lived experience helps them engage angry, fearful, or distrustful parents, and they can explain to parents how the helping system works. When parents have a better understanding of how the system works, they are in a better position to interact with that system in ways that help them get better help.

Family partners are also well positioned to help families make sense of the conflicts that can occur among collaborating helpers. While helpers often focus on the relationship they have with families, there is less emphasis on the relationships helpers have with each other and the positive or negative impact that might have on families. When helpers appreciate each other and work well together, families sense that and generally feel more hopeful. Conversely, when there are difficulties among collaborating helpers, families sense that also, and it can contribute to frustration and hopelessness. As Anthony Irsfeld (personal communication, April 22, 2013), a leading expert in wraparound in Massachusetts, has put it,

> Family partners have a wonderful way of letting families in on the secret that we all are just people with strengths and weaknesses,

mostly trying to do the best we can. I find that family partners can help mitigate the potential negative effects of a system that isn't working well together. Rarely does a helper say to a family, "It's not your fault . . . I just have a hard time dealing with that other worker." What is more likely, in my experience, is that the family picks up on the negativity that no one is acknowledging. When that happens, families are at risk of appearing more defensive or cautious with providers, which then starts a negative cycle where helpers feel frustrated with them. Because we as professionals don't regularly own our part in this, it can lead to an erosion of engagement. In such situations, family partners can help explain to a family. "It's not you, it's the helpers. They are working on getting their act together to be more helpful to you." Family partners have credibility because they are part of the helping system. And most of the time, family partners can then begin to advocate that the helpers "handle their business" with each other so the family can stop worrying about it.

With this in mind, let's move on to some of the ways in which family partners, at their best, position themselves with families in advocacy efforts and the lessons this may hold for the larger helping community.

RELATIONAL STANCE AND ADVOCACY EFFORTS

Consider the follow description of advocacy efforts from a family partner:

> Many of the people we serve are so disempowered. They've been told over and over again that "they can't, they can't, they can't" and then are further criticized when they don't. So, it becomes important to walk through the steps with them. Some of the parents I work with have cognitive difficulties and there are calls they need to make that they struggle with, like calling the phone company to get service restored. I don't tell them to make the call. I don't make the call for them. I tell them we're going to do it together as a conference call. And we plan out ahead of time what needs to happen and how they want to handle it. Then, I'm like a coach in the background to support them in carrying out that plan. And often, I have to remember to step in just enough to help them be successful and stand back enough for them to own that success. Sometimes that's a difficult balance.

Indeed it is. While that balance may be straightforward in theory, it is difficult to put into actual practice. As helpers, we can become caught up in our own desire for a good outcome and overstep to achieve that outcome (e.g., focusing on the short-term goal of getting a mother's phone service restored and losing sight of the longer term goal of helping her expand her capacity to more successfully negotiate life's difficulties). It's important in our efforts to advocate in partnership with people that we "lead from beside," remembering this is their life and our job is to build on their resourcefulness and to interact with them in ways that contribute to their sense of competence and personal agency. It can be a difficult enterprise that requires patience and thoughtfulness, as highlighted in this story from another family partner.

> It's a long process. Parents may start off in the driver's seat with us next to them coaching them and the next day it's like they're in the backseat complaining about how hard it is and encouraging us into the driver's seat. It's hard to not get frustrated with the inevitable setbacks and keep on believing that they can get back to the driver's seat and encouraging them to do that, but that's the job.

POWER DYNAMICS IN WORKING WITH THE LARGER HELPING SYSTEM

Helping work with people normally involves moving through a broad range of some pretty complicated service systems. Let's take a look at some of the common challenges and dilemmas encountered to see how helping workers and people have made it through together. We'll begin with responses to a question posed to multiple workers in home and community settings—What do you find most difficult about working within the larger helping system?

> People don't take me seriously. They think because I'm meeting with people in their homes that I'm somehow less of a professional and have less to offer than them. I've heard things like "How can you call yourself a professional? You don't even have an office." What they don't realize is that it's way harder seeing people on their own turf than in a nice and neat office. I actually know more about people from having seen them in their own environment.

My own outrage about how professionals talk about families. I sit in meetings, particularly when clients are there, and it just feels like torture. They are either ignored or treated like they're in need of some kind of re-education. I alternate between wanting to leave or simply explode and I know neither response is going to be particularly helpful.

Trying to highlight family strengths and having people treat me like I'm some naïve optimist viewing the world through rose-colored lenses. I'm really tired of the eye rolling and scornful glances that my comments seem to provoke.

Do these stories sound familiar? We have experienced these kinds of frustration many times and have heard hundreds of similar stories from other home and community workers. There is a sort of class system of the occupations that spans the spectrum of health and human services. There are distinct power differences among the disciplines of medicine, psychiatry, psychology, social work, nursing, family therapy, counseling, and the rest. Power differences are even more pronounced when expanded to include workers in outreach, home health, child protection, residential care, case management, and other home and community settings. We may have created a situation where the higher the helping professional is in the service hierarchy, the less intimate contact the helper actually has with the people served. What kind of message does this send?

In any system with significant differences in power and authority, distinct dynamics and issues of privilege arise where people holding more privilege are often less aware of the experiences of people with less privilege. Health and human service systems are no exception. Communications within these systems are influenced by preexisting race, class, gender, sexual orientation, and other power dynamics. It is inevitable that interactions between helpers, the people we serve, and other health and human service system partners are all influenced in one way or another by dynamics of privilege. Consider the following.

An esteemed, older white male family therapist comes to do a consultation at a local agency. A young Latina woman presents a family with a teenage boy who has struggled with depression and is on a slew of medications. At one point, the consultant asks why this boy is on so much medication. The outreach worker responds, "I don't know. That's what his psychiatrist put him on." The consultant asks her why she hasn't confronted the psychiatrist on this fact. She responds that the psychiatrist doesn't return her calls and the consultant instructs her to call the psychiatrist and let him know that the consultant has determined the boy is over-medicated. She nods in agreement, but then over beers that evening with co-workers announces that the consultant has to be crazy to suggest she call out a psychiatrist who serves as the medical director of her agency. Her co-workers laugh and order another round.

Here we have a man with greater sociocultural and professional influence instructing a woman with significantly less socially sanctioned power to make a phone call with no awareness of the potential consequences for her. While she laughed it off with fellow workers after the consultation, she later described the embarrassment and frustration of feeling tongue-tied in the moment. The consultant came away believing his instruction had been successful. He had no way to know that not only did the consultation not resonate for the helping worker but also that she walked away with absolutely no intention of following through. Patterns of "pseudocompliance" emerge in care systems where communication is overly formal and often superficial. Professional conversations like these create a predictable response from people in a one-down position. The outreach worker very likely has a much better understanding than the consultant of actual skills needed to successfully negotiate her particular larger service system dynamics. If we do not intentionally design care systems that are open and respectful, professional privilege and credentialing can too easily suppress the needed perspective of home and community workers. An overly narrow view limits our accumulated wisdom and hampers our ability to move forward together. It can also create destructive self-marginalization where helping workers come to doubt their own perspective, losing sight of insights that are only obtainable through collaborative work in a natural home and community environment.

The consultant's lack of awareness of the actual effects of his "intervention" highlights the responsibility we all have as helping workers to consider potential disempowering effects of our actions. This includes many of our taken-for-granted professional practices, like how we talk about people and families. Consider this description.

> A young worker sits in a school team meeting feeling completely lost in a sea of jargon she doesn't understand. She complains to her supervisor who comforts her and then wonders how the mother who was also in that meeting might have felt. The worker asks this mother about that and is told, "It was terrible. I had no idea what you all were saying and it was very clear to me that there was no place for me in that meeting. I felt like a horrible mother and went home and cried for the rest of the afternoon."

The professionals in the meeting had no intention of dismantling this mother's confidence in her own parenting. This was simply their way of speaking in meetings and this kind of "professional speak" is pretty common. But helping workers who are aware of and witness such unintended negative effects often become frustrated, angry, and just unsure of how to respond. Family partners have played an important role in helping service teams reflect on the effects of common practices and develop more respectful and responsive ways of interacting with people and families. They are sometimes vocal in challenging condescending talk. But it is a role that can take quite a toll. It can be sort of like listening to a racist, sexist, or homophobic joke and blowing the whistle while people all around are laughing and having fun. It takes timing and skill along with considerable strength of conviction.

Helping workers committed to a collaborative approach often experience special challenges within the larger helping system. Their commitment to strengths-based, accountable partnerships can collide with more traditional treatment approaches that focus on deficits, elevate professional wisdom, and often encourage helpers to feel responsible *for* the people they serve rather than responsible *to* them (Madsen, 2006, 2007a, b). We can draw from a cross-cultural metaphor and think of these different approaches as representing diverse helping cultures. Unfortunately, the dominant theme of professionalism usually favors a more traditional approach at the expense of collaboration. Although this seems to be changing, the ideas and principles of a more collaborative helping culture can still be seen as weird, naive, and perhaps even downright silly. Home and community workers too often experience the perception of their contribution as being somehow less professional. These biases about legitimacy that pervade assumptions about what counts and what doesn't are clearly evolving throughout helping cultures. As health and human service payment systems move in the direction of performance-based contracting and related reforms, a more collaborative, person-centered approach to health and well-being is growing. As a field, we've both come a long way and still have a ways to go.

DILEMMAS IN ADVOCACY EFFORTS

Let's examine some of the challenges in advocacy efforts and different ways workers have responded to them. We'll begin with an examination of two common problematic interactions that can develop between helping workers committed to these ideas and their more traditional colleagues.

The first is a minimize/maximize pattern where attempts to highlight strengths and resourcefulness are perceived by other professionals as minimizing problems, thereby inviting attempts to counterbalance that with an impressive accounting of pathology. This is a common experience for helping workers operating from a strengths-based perspective. As they work with people to identify strengths and assets, they are inclined to share their perspective with others within the larger helping system. Other professionals who are predisposed by training, professional culture, or both, may have a very different experience of the same people and can experience strengths-based helpers as "starry-eyed optimists who minimize real problems." In turn, the strengths-based helpers may experience more traditional helpers as "blinded by a disease model." The resulting polarization ends up confirming the worst of both stereotypes and inadvertently entrenching respective worldviews.

A second potential problematic pattern in working with traditional professionals is an instruct/resist pattern. Attempts to share a strengths-based perspective with other collaborating helpers may be heard as stories told by crusading missionaries. This can lead to an experience of collaborative helpers as "holier than thou" and contribute to an escalating interaction that again rigidifies respective perspectives and undercuts shared work. Identifying these patterns is the first step to responding differently and developing more constructive interactions. Our work with other professionals, as well as with the people we're helping, needs to be grounded in strengths-based, collaborative partnerships. The attitude we bring to our work with other helpers is every bit as important as our relationship with people served. When we find ourselves in conflict with other helpers, it is important to respect their knowledge, honor their intentions, and find ways to view their perspective as part of a larger picture.

Responding to Advocacy Dilemmas and Developing Relational Connection With Other Helpers

We turn now to the experiences of a rural home and community-centered organization that has moved from the margins to become an integral part of the local health and human service delivery system. The organization has been working in a remote Appalachian region for over 20 years. Over that time, they have evolved to play a critical role across multiple helping systems. Here are some reflections from a supervisor, Terri, on how they've accomplished that.

> We hung in there doing the work year after year. Our work stands on its own because we repeatedly took on the hardest situations. In fact, we consistently asked for that. We'd say to referral sources, "Give us your hardest, most complicated families. That's who we work with." And that's what we do. We go out and meet people in their natural environment and get to know them in a holistic way—their likes and dislikes, their hopes and dreams, the everyday stuff they encounter. We know the people we serve in a very intimate way and over time we've built a reputation as people who "are in the know."

And how have you built that reputation?

> We just kept doing the work and talking to other helpers about the work we were doing. We were good at letting people know what we were doing and at this point, the rest of the helping system has come to know us, trust us, and count on us. We make a point of building relationships, not only with the people we serve, but also with other helpers and with the people who fund us. It's all about relationship.

Similarly, a group of family partners in a wraparound program in an urban setting began as a group of outspoken minority mothers with a reputation as fierce advocates who you didn't want to mess with. As they gained more and more respect within their state, they were utilized as consultants in the process of expanding the use of family partners in wraparound programs across the state. Here, Yvette describes one of the ways in which she helped a child psychiatrist reflect on some of his taken-for-granted assumptions.

> I remember him saying, "I feel like I love this kid more than his mom because his mom wants him out of the house and I think he needs to be home. How can she really want her kid to be removed?" And, I was able to sit there and help him see that it wasn't that this mother didn't love her son but that she was tired and dragged down and she needed him to be safe. If putting him in a lock-up would accomplish that, it would be okay with her. The psychiatrist could say he loved that kid more than his mom because he didn't understand where she was coming from. And I felt proud about helping him see things a bit differently.

How did you do that?

> I did it in a way that didn't blame or insult him. Even though I might have been thinking "How dare you say that," I didn't say it. Because I've lived through similar things, I was able to say it in a way that helped him understand that it was okay for a mother to feel that and say that. And I did it making eye contact and speaking from my experience rather than speaking from some "know it all" place.

And what was important for you in doing it that way?

> Well, I've had to learn to check my own feelings at the door, especially anger, and bring into the room a more gentle and softer side of me and get that across. I want to stay very clear about what my purpose is and how I can engage other professionals in ways that are really going to help the people I serve. I say to myself, "This meeting is not for me." It is for the family and how can I relate to other helpers in ways that keep the family at the center of what I do.
>
> I also use my own experiences and connect them with what parents are saying to emphasize their points. So, rather than saying, "The mother is very angry," I might say, "I remember when I was going through this, I was very angry." I can talk about my own experience and use that as a way to advocate for parents. Using my own experience allows me to have it be on me rather than on the mother.

The use of personal stories by family partners in their interactions with both families and other helpers is built into the role of family partner.

It can raise some interesting dilemmas for them about which stories to use and which to hold back. We think Ellen Walnum (2007, p. 6) draws a distinction between personal and private stories that can be very helpful here.

> Within my work, I also take care to separate "personal" and "private" stories. In my conversations with children and adults, I am proudly sharing personal stories from my life. But I am not sharing my private stories. For instance, the particular experiences I had with my mother are private stories; they are between her and me, and I have shared them only with my husband, my son, and a few close friends and colleagues. All I tell other people is that my mother said and did things that mothers are not supposed to do. I think that is enough. This distinction between personal and private is an important one. In meeting with others, I am always aware that they too should have a choice as to what they want to share and with whom. In the professional world, it seems as if personal stories and private stories get blurred and because of this workers are often afraid to share any of their personal stories. They see the sharing of personal stories as "unprofessional." I don't see it this way and I think much more thought needs to go into this. Experience consultants have a lot to offer in this regard.

Let's return to the challenges that family partners encounter in larger system meetings. Janice, another family partner, highlights some of the dilemmas for her in responding to objectifying and pathologizing language in wraparound meetings.

> We often have to battle out our own feelings about how parents are treated because it reminds us of how we were treated. We have to stay very clear about how we can be most helpful for the particular parent in that room at that moment. When we're doing wraparound meetings, we need to keep these other professionals at the table. We can't go along with business as usual, but we also can't afford to offend them and have them drop out of the process. And that can be a tricky tightrope to walk.

Another family partner adds,

> We're really in a position of respectful mediators. Because many times, let's be honest, we're working with families who don't

like the helpers in their lives and helpers who don't like the families. And we can be in the middle and help them get to know each other in respectful ways and help them each find ways to talk to the other. So, we're kind of like some combination of mediators and translators, trying to help them work collaboratively.

And this process of mediating and negotiating, how do you do that in meetings with families and other helpers?

We work very closely with the families so that their voice is brought to the table in a way that is respected and heard. We try to make sure that we're not just going through the motions— check, check, check, meeting's done—but are really making sure that we take time to consider what parents are saying and what the meetings are like for them.

I think families often feel as if providers are blaming and shaming them, essentially conveying the idea that your kid is the way she is because of you. And that's not true. Their kid is the way she is because of the problems that have come into her life and we need to keep a focus on how we can support them in the process.

They have found this shift from focusing on what is happening in the present and what needs to change to focusing on what could be different in the future and how helpers can assist in that process to be very helpful in these situations. Here are some other ways they have worked to more actively involve parents in meetings:

From Janice: When I see a mother sinking, I'll often ask her how she's doing in front of the team to open up the door for something different to happen. So, I might say in front of the team, "Mom, are you feeling frustrated?" and if she says yes, I'll ask her, "What can we do to help you in this situation? What would be the best thing for us to be talking about now? How can we help make things better? How can we make a difference?" This is a way to get us back on track.

From Yvette: I think when parents are in a place of despair and see us acknowledging their pain and advocating for them, they can feel like there's someone at this table who is supporting me and that gives them hope in dealing with their larger situation. It makes them less alone and conveys to other helpers that we can do better than this.

Family partners' roles sometimes position them in ways that offer them opportunities to draw on their own experiences to help other parents and relate to collaborating workers. Outreach workers are in a different role and so let's look at some of the strategies they've developed to bridge how they relate to families and other workers. We'll begin with Terri who we heard from previously.

> We're kind of like chameleons in a good sense of that word. We fit to the environment we're in. When we're out with families, we dress and talk casually, and when we're in professional settings, we fit to that. At the same time, we are always trying to be real and relate directly to whoever we are with at that moment. We ask other helpers about their personal lives and make a point of getting to know them as real human beings.
>
> And when we're in settings where the people we work with and other helpers are all in the same room, we make a point of letting people served know ahead of time what they can expect from us and make sure they feel like we have their back. So, we might say, "There's likely to be a lot of jargon in this meeting and if that's unfamiliar to you, give me a look and I'll ask about it." We're all about fitting ourselves to the situation we're in and helping the people we serve negotiate those same situations as best they can.
>
> At the same time, with other professionals we work extra hard to keep alive a sense of when all is said and done, we are part of the same team. We reach out to them in the same way that we reach out to families. We have to realize that the outside agencies are our clients also.

Terri's comments highlight the importance of the attitude with which we approach other helpers. While this is easy to suggest, it is more challenging to put into practice. Here is Terri's response to the question of how she stays grounded in a constructive attitude despite considerable frustration with other helpers.

> I think we all are really committed to helping the people we serve get to a better place and I think we recognize that if we are not cooperative, engaging of, and serving to other agencies, even

as frustrating as some may be, it ultimately hurts our clients. We all have our challenges and particular people or agencies that drive us crazy, but we just keep plugging away.

One of the things that helped this team in engaging other helpers is an appreciation of the larger context in which we all work. Here are further comments from them based on this realization.

> From Keith: While there's support for benevolence for people served, there's more license for righteous anger and indignation for injustice by the court or Child Protective Services or the housing authority, the landlord, etc. We have a cultural predisposition for anger. Advocacy is laden with license for anger against systems and it's not helpful. It works to the detriment of the people we serve. So here's the thing. These helpers are people as well and we're in a relationship with them as clearly as we are in a relationship with people served. We know them over time, we're working with them, we're trying to get along in a world of social relationships. To me, it's the same.
>
> From Terri: It's almost the natural order of things. There has to be a little tension in order for the different systems to work together. The court has a serious job to do; CPS has a serious job to do.
>
> From Darlene: One of the things that I try to help people with is an understanding that there is harshness in these agencies and these systems, but we still have to deal with them. People served can't just say, "I don't want your services. Screw it. I'm leaving." That's not going to work. You won't get anywhere throwing your hands up and walking out.
>
> From Keith: Part of the tension is that systems are designed in ways that people working there are licensed with obligations for enforcement and surveillance and rule keeping and all that stuff and that's their job. And it does form their participation in relationships. Another problem here is grinding poverty. We're talking about counties that don't have money for lice problems. They don't have the money to keep their county offices heated in winter. The problem here is grinding poverty and a patchwork service system.

This appreciation of the larger context helps keep us focused on the best hopes and shared goals for people served throughout the helping system. While different helpers may be operating from different assumptions, we are all operating within a system with significant flaws in its ability to respond to people in need. From here, let's examine some innovative ways to support people served in finding a voice amid the chaos of helping efforts.

HELPING PEOPLE MORE EFFECTIVELY ADVOCATE FOR THEMSELVES

We have focused here on the importance of three things. The first is how helpers position themselves in interactions with people, holding an awareness of how people might experience those interactions and how that experience might contribute to the development of particular life stories. The second is how helpers can engage in advocacy efforts in partnership with people served and respond to the larger helping system in a connected rather than adversarial fashion. And the third is the need to develop organizational structures that encourage more respectful and responsive ways of interacting with people and families, rather than simply relying on the efforts of individuals.

One effort that brings these three things together is the Right Question Project, founded by Dan Rothstein and Luz Santana (2011).[1] Their work represents an effort to help people advocate for themselves and actively participate in the help provided to them by formulating and asking questions using specific criteria for accountable decision making. They began their work in Lawrence, Massachusetts, working with low-income parents in a dropout prevention program. In the process of trying to engage these parents, they learned that many were not participating in their children's education because they "didn't even know what to ask." They began by trying to develop questions for parents to ask and eventually moved to teaching people how to formulate their own questions. For the past 20 years, they have been designing and refining a way to do this as simply and effectively as possible. While their work began in education and literacy contexts, they have subsequently expanded it to public agencies, social services, mental health, and health care. The heart of their work is developing frameworks for accountable decision making and helping people to formulate and ask questions about issues of importance to them. They've come to believe that all people, no matter their level of income or education, can use these skills to help themselves, their families, and their communities.

Their work involves aiding people who are seeking services to develop their capacity to ask questions of workers that clarify their hopes for help and assisting them to become more active participants in the helping process. There is a particular focus on how decisions are being made, the criteria being used in those decisions, and what role they can take in decisions about their care. Across a variety of situations, they found that when people seeking help entered with some clearly articulated questions about the help provided to them based on their own hopes, the same people became more active and empowered participants in their own care.

The Right Question Project is consistent with our ideas about Collaborative Helping. Assisting people to become active participants in helping efforts designed for them has great potential for all helping workers across health and human services. For example, before wraparound meetings, family partners could help parents formulate questions that they want to bring to the meeting. Similarly, workers in health care, child protection, residential, mental health, juvenile justice, and pretty much all other home and community contexts could similarly have these kinds of conversations as preparation for any important meeting that puts helping professionals and the people they serve in a room together.

In addition, the three components of the framework for accountable decision making (the *process* for making a decision, the *role* people served play in that process, and the *reason* for the final decision that affects them) could easily be incorporated into any team meeting in order to create clear and transparent meeting structures that are accountable to people served. We have talked repeatedly about definitional ceremonies and the idea that our meetings with people have the potential to invite them into particular experiences of self that may lift them up and carry them forward or drag them down and inadvertently convince them of their inadequacy and continued need for additional services. The idea of enabling people to actively formulate questions that keep helping professionals accountable to the people they serve represents a radical reconstruction of the helping process.

IN THE END, IT'S STILL WALKING AND TALKING

We began this chapter by returning to a guiding metaphor for our work of "walking and talking"—concrete assistance paired with thoughtful conversation. We compared some of the differences between working on professional turf (in an office) and working on family turf (in people's homes and communities). In this different context, a number of traditional notions about "professional boundaries" play out in very different ways. One apt summary of this came from a worker who drew a distinction between "boundary lines" and "boundary ropes" that can be tightened or loosened depending on the situation and the relationship that exists. This more flexible definition of boundaries creates opportunities but also poses challenges and dilemmas, and we featured stories of some of the ways in which different helpers have negotiated these situations. With the expansion of home and community work, we are seeing new developments in professional ethics that are grounded in an appreciation of strengths, a preference for partnership, and a commitment to cultural responsiveness and accountability (being responsible *to* people served rather than being responsible *for* them). It will be exciting to see these developments continue to unfold.

We also brought in the contributions of family partners and highlighted Ellen Walnum's consideration of this role as that of an "experience consultant." Family partners hold great potential to connect with people through a deep experiential understanding of what they are going through. They can also profoundly help health and human service agencies develop more sensitivity to those experiences and provide help in which people feel better heard and more assured that they matter.

Finally, we highlighted a number of important considerations in advocacy efforts. It is crucial to ensure that we advocate alongside people, contributing to and supporting their efforts, instead of falling into simply speaking on their behalf. We heard from multiple perspectives about the importance of connected advocacy in which we stand with the people we serve and maintain connections with the larger helping systems in which they are operating. Hopefully, their stories provide starter dough for further ideas about how we might continue to do this. In conclusion, the material covered in this chapter may lead to a rather simple point: People do better when they can get help that is relevant in the context of their own world, encourages their active participation, and comes across as really interested, genuine, and clear.

NOTE

1. The Right Question Project has grown into the Right Question Institute. For more information about their work, please consult their website at www.rightquestion.org.

CHAPTER 8

Sustainable Helping

We have laid out a broad framework for helping that grounds our work in a spirit of respect, connection, curiosity, and hope. We've examined an overall approach to this work and delved into the ways in which this is put into practice on a daily basis. This chapter looks at supervisory and organizational practices that can sustain these efforts. We discuss ways that supervisors can use Collaborative Helping maps to support their efforts to enhance collaborative practice. Then, we move to an organizational level to examine leadership styles and institutional practices that can support collaborative ways of working.

USING COLLABORATIVE HELPING MAPS TO ENHANCE SUPERVISION

Collaborative Helping maps can also be used in supervisory conversations about individuals and families. They provide a vehicle for supervisors and workers to collectively think their way through complex situations. While these maps were originally designed for use with families and have had beneficial effects on helping relationships, we have found that their use in supervision also enhances supervisory relationships and can have transformative effects on workers. Their repeated use over time helps workers develop "habits of thought" that can bring more rigor and discipline into their work. They can introduce workers to new ways of thinking about vision, obstacles, supports, and plans. And finally, they can assist supervisors in helping workers draw on supports and shift their own relationship to obstacles to work more effectively with families. This section introduces an adaptation of Collaborative Helping maps for supervision and briefly examines one way they have been used in supervisory consultations. While supervision in community agencies often serves many functions, we focus here on the use of these maps to organize conversations about more effective work with individuals and families. A Collaborative Helping map adapted for a supervisory context is shown in Figure 8.1, with sample questions to highlight each section. Let's walk through the map, highlighting the purpose of each section, and then illustrate how it was used in a supervisory consult.

The *Purpose and Context* section of this supervisory map is an opportunity to clarify and align worker and supervisor hopes and purposes for the supervisory meeting.[1] Taking the time to gain agreement about purpose is actually an investment that saves time in the long run. For example, how many times have you found yourself in a meeting wondering, "What are we doing here?" How might the meeting have gone differently if you had a clear sense of its purpose? Clarifying hopes and purposes generally leads to a better meeting. Supervision in home- and community-oriented service organizations often takes place in a pressure cooker of conflicting demands that creates a multitasking frenzy. Context questions such as "What might be getting in the way of you being fully present here today?" and "In the midst of everything else going on, how can we make this time as useful as possible for you?" acknowledge that context and provide a way for workers and supervisors to carve out a small space for reflection. The final question about stakeholders seeks to ensure that we have the right people in the room for the conversation we wish to have. Many times this is not possible, but inquiring about the possibility acknowledges some of the contextual realities we face together.

The *Introduction of the Person or Family* section is an opportunity to learn about people in a way that highlights elements of competence, connection, and hope. In a counseling context, case presentations often begin in a fashion similar to "Patient is a 30-year-old borderline female with significant difficulties regulating affect." As a reader, how would you prefer to be introduced to a group of strangers who had significant influence over your life? How might an introduction like the one here impact your own "affect regulation?" In a spirit of "contact before content," we prefer to get to know people in a helping relationship as three-dimensional human beings before entering into an investigation of their difficulties. We believe this holds true whether we are actually meeting them or simply having a conversation about them. Asking

FIGURE 8.1   **OUTLINE FOR SUPERVISORY COLLABORATIVE HELPING MAP**

Purpose and Context of the Supervisory Conversation
• Purpose—What do you hope to get out of us talking today about this? • Context—Is there anything that might get in the way of you being able to focus in on this conversation? • Stakeholders—Is there anyone else who is not here who should be part of this conversation?
Introduction of the Person or Family
• Who are the members of this family and their network? • How do you think they might like you to introduce them to us? • What is it like for you working with them? (What do you like about working with them? What is hard about working with them?)
Agreed-Upon Focus
• In 25 words or less, what might different members of this family say their work with you is heading toward? • What might other helpers involved with the family say? What would you say? • What similarities and differences do you notice in these different descriptions? • On a scale of 0–10, how would family members, you, and other helpers rate progress toward these goals? • What similarities and differences do you notice in these different descriptions?

Obstacles	**Supports**
• What might different family members and other helpers say gets in way of things going better toward agreed-upon focus? • What would you say gets in the way of things going better toward agreed-upon focus? • What similarities and differences do you notice? • How have these obstacles gotten in the way of your agreed-upon focus and what problematic effects have they had on your work together?	• What might family members and others helpers say has contributed to things going as well as they have toward agreed-upon focus? • What would you say has contributed to things going as well as they have toward agreed-upon focus? • What similarities and differences do you notice? • How have these supports contributed to your agreed-upon focus and what beneficial effects have they had on your work together?

Plan
• Based on what you've heard yourself saying about vision, obstacles, and supports, what do you think is the next step to help this family draw on supports to address obstacles to "live into" vision? • Who will do what, when, and with whom? • Who else needs to be involved?

Reflection on the Supervisory Conversation	
Plus	**Delta**
• What went well in our meeting today that you'd like to see us continue in future meetings?	• What could we do differently to make this better in the future?

helpers how people served might like to be introduced humanizes them. And the final question in this section helps get a sense of the helping relationship and gives workers an opportunity to talk about both what they appreciate and find difficult in that relationship. This is important to make supervisory conversations responsive to helping workers and to get a sense of the emotionally laden responses that often end up implicitly hijacking supervisory conversations.

The *Agreed-Upon Focus* section elicits a proactive focus for the work of helping from different perspectives and encourages a comparison that facilitates shared vision. The scaling question allows a mutual assessment of where things are currently and sets up an examination of obstacles and supports to both build on emerging progress and address challenges.

The *Obstacles* and *Supports* sections of the Collaborative Helping map encourage workers to identify obstacles and supports at individual, relational, and sociocultural levels. When applied to supervision, we can shift these levels to include obstacles and supports at a family level (which would include individual, relational, and sociocultural levels), obstacles and supports at a family-helper level (interactions that have developed between workers and the people they serve as well as the broader professional and sociocultural contexts in which those interactions occur), and obstacles and supports at a helping level (a worker's negative or positive emotional reactions to a family, beliefs or stories about a family and their possibilities, and the broader taken-for-granted professional and cultural assumptions and practices that may support these various reactions and stories). We can conceptualize these three levels of obstacles as concentric circles as highlighted in Figure 8.2.

FIGURE 8.2   **THREE LEVELS TO CONSIDER IN SUPERVISION**

Three Levels to Consider

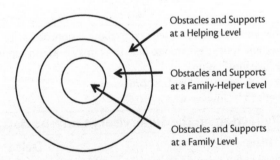

Obstacles and Supports
at a Helping Level

Obstacles and Supports
at a Family-Helper Level

Obstacles and Supports
at a Family Level

The *Plan* section asks helping workers to put the pieces together and in a way that positions the supervisor as an ally to support rather than to supplant worker thinking. There is obviously room here for supervisors to add to workers' ideas, but it is critical to first elicit worker thinking and then proceed with further ideas in an additive fashion. It is also important to keep this area concretely focused on action planning organized by practical clarifying questions.

The final *Reflection* section encourages continuing feedback and shared learning. The *Plus* (+) column seeks to build on what went well. The *Delta* (Δ or the Greek symbol for change) column seeks to elicit what could go better. This extends an investigation of "What was good and not so good?" to a more constructive "What was good and what could be better?" It elicits useful feedback for supervisors, encourages shared learning, and models a process for workers in their own interactions with people and families.

In order to illustrate this, consider the following supervisory consult: The Johnson family is a working-class African-American family that has a long involvement with Child Protective Services because of concerns about neglect primarily due to the mother's substance use. The parents are currently divorced and the three young children (2, 3, and 4) are living with their father and have been doing well until the most recent incident when the father was arrested for a DUI (his first) with the three children in the car. He took responsibility for what he called "a mistake in judgment" and he and the CPS worker have developed a plan they are both comfortable with to ensure that the children will not be put into a similar situation again in the future. They are served by an office in which the worker, supervisor, and manager are all African-American. There are significant protective concerns in the broader office about this family due to the long history with substances. This concern has been exacerbated by a recent phone call from a neighbor to a local African-American politician who is putting significant pressure on the department to "come down hard" on the family and take a strong "no tolerance" stance. The manager in the office has increasing concerns about the situation and there is an increasing polarization developing between the worker and the manager in which the supervisor feels caught.

Susan is a child protective supervisor who sought a consultation about this situation from Bill. When asked what she hoped to get out of the consultation, Susan responded, "This is a case where there are differences of opinion about how to move forward among the worker, me as the supervisor, and our manager and I'd like to find a way to better address that. We have a lot of outside pressure on this case and I'd like to sort out how we can do good work in that context." Susan gave a brief description of the family, and we moved into an examination of obstacles and supports for good work in the face of outside pressures. Because the purpose of the consultation was to clarify how the team might best work with this family, Bill focused on obstacles to and supports for good work at an office level, rather than focusing on the family or the worker. When asked how the differences of opinion were playing out, Susan described the manager as much more worried about the situation than the worker and expressed a concern that conversations about the family were becoming increasingly stuck. We traced out an overly protective/overly harsh pattern in which the manager saw the worker as being too "soft" with the family and the worker saw the manager as being too "hard" with the family. We can think of this interaction as a series of mutual invitations in which one person's actions invite a particular response from the other and that response in turn invites a counterresponse. The interaction occurred in a broader context of outside pressure that fueled the manager's concerns and in turn exacerbated the worker's sense of others "meddling with his work." When asked about the effects of this pattern on their work and relationships in the office, Susan worried about the potential for escalating polarization and described herself as caught in the middle.

It was not an unusual situation for them to have differences of opinion amid significant outside pressures, so Bill inquired about other "different, but similar" situations that might hold relevant lessons. That led into a discussion of how they had managed political pressures in the past. The worker, supervisor, and manager were all good at advocating for their own position, while listening to others' perspectives. When asked how they had successfully resolved differences in the past, Susan described the use of the same mapping process occurring with her in this consultation. As the consultation moved into the plan section, obstacles and supports were identified, and Susan was asked what she thought needed to happen next. She thought a moment and replied that she wanted to have a meeting with the father, worker, herself, and manager. She would facilitate a Collaborative Helping map process with all of them. She thought that would help them examine different perspectives in a transparent process and move forward thoughtfully. It was agreed and logistics were discussed. From here, let's expand our focus from a supervisory to an organizational level.

BUILDING INSTITUTIONAL STRUCTURES THAT SUPPORT COLLABORATION

Let's examine organizational practices that encourage respect, connection, curiosity, and hope within organizations and across helping systems. We'll begin with a story from Shaheer, who became the new director of an established, large residential program for children that was highlighted in Chapter 4. Shaheer entered with a commitment to building a family-centered program and began by meeting with staff members and talking with them about the things they did well and the things they hoped to do better. Based on those conversations, his program developed three core principles and values that they called their ABCs. Here is his description.

> *A* is for *Accountability*. Across the board, everybody felt like we could do better at being accountable to kids, to families, and to each other. So, for example, there were times when we would make a mistake around a pass and the parent maybe didn't get to see their kid because we screwed up on something. In the past, there wouldn't even necessarily be an apology for that. It was like, "Your kid's in a residential program, stuff happens. Sorry." But now, we're accountable. If we screwed up, we need to own that and say, "I'm really sorry. That was an oversight on our part and we'll do our best to make sure that never happens again." And so, accountability meant just owning that to a family and then working to correct it.
>
> The *B* in the ABCs stands for *Believing in the possibility of success* for every kid and family. In the past, we got so bogged down in the histories of these kids and what we heard from referral sources. To shift that, we decided to believe that every kid and family could be successful and tried to operate with that assumption in mind. So, regardless of what we were told and regardless of what we saw, we held to the idea that change is possible and hope exists. Practicing that belief made a difference and I think it came across to kids and families in how we interacted with them.
>
> And the *C* is for *Collaboration* with kids, families, and other helping professionals. It meant we work with families; we don't

act upon families. We get their feedback. An example of that is our nursing department. When kids come here, we're responsible for their entire health care. In the past, health assistants would just take kids to the local clinic. And I thought, "That doesn't really feel collaborative to me. Do we ask the parents where they would prefer their kid to be seen? Do they want to come? Should we be asking or encouraging them to come?" That was not something that was well received because it was easier for us to just do it. But eventually our staff came around and that's what we do now. So, anytime a kid has an appointment, we call the family and tell them, "Here's what's going on. We'd like to schedule an appointment. What do you think about that? If that makes sense, do you want to come along?" We don't want to be in a position of taking care of their kid; we want them to take care of their kid. That was a big shift for people.

As the ABCs became an accepted norm and part of ongoing conversations in the program, they expanded their efforts to weave these principles into the fabric of organizational culture through a variety of institutional practices. This included efforts to change their paperwork, staff evaluations, and clinical discussion formats. We examine each of these efforts next.

Rethinking Paperwork

Paperwork in home and community agencies is an interesting phenomenon. Sometimes it can feel like an unfortunate necessity, completed at the last moment before an audit. Sometimes it almost requires the sort of unkind descriptions of the people we serve that workers may be justifiably reluctant to show them. For helping workers committed to a collaborative approach, the traditional assessment and planning format can be a real hindrance. Historically, assessments have begun with a description of the problem and its precipitants, then an examination of the history that led up to the problem, then current functioning and relevant medical information, then risk factors and mental status, and finally a formulation leads to and justifies a particular diagnosis. Service planning follows in much the same manner. We believe it is possible to revamp paperwork in ways that support and enhance collaborative work.

The challenge of recasting paperwork may seem difficult given the demands of licensure, certification, and accreditation. But it is not impossible, and rapid system change affecting all public health and human services seems to be creating a unique opening. Madsen (2004, 2007a, b) has devoted extensive attention to formats for assessments, collaborative treatment plans, and termination / consolidation summaries that fit licensing requirements. While space does not allow us to replicate those outlines in detail here, readers who are interested might want to consult those works, which discuss this in depth and offer generic forms for such paperwork. Many agencies across different contexts have used these materials to develop locally adapted paperwork that supports collaborative work in their particular contexts. In fact, the integration of behavioral health with primary health care and the creation of person-centered health homes combine with requirements for electronic health records to potentially open doors for creativity. Though this may seem counterintuitive at first, the migration of data through the Internet and into the "cloud" is making possible broad learning communities where a new kind of collaborative innovation is possible. But we must embrace the moment together or bureaucracy will simply replicate itself in a new and even more unforgiving automated environment.

As paperwork moves into data clouds, we expect new alliances to form that support the transformation of old style disease-oriented documentation toward a new way of doing service business that better supports the general health and well-being of people and communities. We trust that Collaborative Helping can be a part of the change process. We can use assessments and treatment plans to organize collaborative efforts around a shared vision. Learning about the importance of this vision for individuals and families makes the work more relevant to them and keeps our work focused on their hopes and desires. Focusing on supports as contributory factors to that vision highlights resourcefulness. Describing obstacles in ways that separate people from problems has some extremely beneficial possibilities that can be supported by assessments and service plans designed along these lines.

Rethinking Staff and Program Evaluations

Another way to sustain collaborative ways of helping is by building key organizing principles into staff and program evaluations. As an example, the residential program we described built their ABCs into employee performance evaluations. They broke down the ABCs into specific goals and then developed a series of objectives, particular to each job description, to operationalize them. As one example, here's how the Accountability goals were structured for a classroom teacher position:

> **Goal:** Accountability:_____ will be accountable to kids, families, and staff/peers.
>
> **Objective 1:_____** will develop individualized learning goals in partnership with each student, their family, and the teaching team. Goals will be approved by the student, family, and team prior to implementation.
>
> **Objective 2:_____** will participate actively during weekly team meetings. They will invite children and families to meetings when their child's progress is scheduled to be discussed and this will be documented in the educational record.

They used a SMART format (Specific, Measurable, Achievable, Relative, and Timely) to develop the goals and objectives. At the same time, recognizing that how a program treats staff will be reflected in how staff in turn treats people seeking help, they also integrated workers' personal and professional aspirations and goals into evaluations as well. As Shaheer put it,

> Supervisors and managers were expected to have professional development plans with the staff or, at a minimum, offer that to them as a way to encourage the larger concept that a learning organization is better equipped to serve the infinite complexities of the people we work with. Obviously, you can't legislate strengths-based, collaborative practice like you can't legislate common sense. However, leaders can be clear about how strengths-based collaborative practice becomes operationalized and can set and monitor expectations so that they become integrated into the day-to-day mechanics of the program.

Moving from staff evaluation to program evaluation, we can organize this process in a way that helps agencies become more accountable to the people they serve. One example of such efforts is the Outcome Rating Scale and the Session Rating Scale developed by Barry Duncan, Scott Miller, and Jackie Sparks. These two simple, user-friendly scales take about a minute each to complete at the end of meetings between helpers and people served. The Outcome Rating Scale (ORS; Miller, Duncan, Brown, Sparks, & Claud, 2003) asks people to evaluate how they're doing in their lives in terms of personal, interpersonal, social, and overall well-being. The Session Rating Scale (SRS; Duncan et al., 2003) asks people to evaluate how helping efforts are going in terms of factors known to be related to effective help (the degree to which people feel heard, understood, and respected; the degree to which the work is focused on what they deem important; the degree to which they feel the helper's approach is a good fit for them; and the degree to which encounters feel right for them). Through completing these scales, people seeking help are invited to become active participants in the outcome measurement process. The scales provide ongoing immediate feedback to helpers as well as openings for conversations about how things are going in helping efforts. While these scales were originally developed for therapy sessions, they have been adapted and applied across a variety of outreach and residential contexts.

At a program level, we can also draw on measures such as the Beach Center Family-Professional Partnership Scale (Blue-Banning, Summers, Nelson, Frankland, & Beegle, 2004). These scales ask people served to rate staff members on a series of collaborative, family-centered behaviors. Some examples of these ratings would include "my child's service provider builds on my child's strengths, my child's service provider shows respect for my family's values and beliefs, my child's service provider is honest even when he or she has bad news, etc." Each of the efforts described here provides concrete ways that organizations can actively support enhanced collaboration with the people they serve. We offer these examples to both alert you as a reader to some interesting efforts and to convey a direction that these and other similar efforts might take.

Rethinking Clinical Discussion Formats

Let's take a look at one example of a structure for bringing the voices of people served into ongoing conversations about them (Madsen, 1996, 2004, 2007a, b). The family voice format is a process for organizing consultations, group supervisions, or any meeting where helpers are talking about people served when they are not present. While we believe that people should always have the right to attend any meeting about them, this is not always possible. This format has one team member sit off to the side and listen to the discussion in the role of a particular person or family member being discussed. At the end of the discussion, the person in the role of the "family voice" is interviewed in role about their experience of the discussion. Questions might include examples such as:

- What was this process like for you and what reactions did you have to it?
- Were there parts of this conversation that were helpful to you? How did that impact you?
- Were there parts of this conversation that were not helpful? How did that impact you?
- If there were negative effects, how could we have had the discussion in a way that addressed difficult issues and yet did not have those effects?

Following that interview, the group briefly discusses their experience of the process and what members would like to take away from it.

The family voice format is a process that invites workers in professional settings to reflect on the real effects of taken-for-granted ways of talking about people. Based on the assumption that how we talk about people outside of their presence shapes how we talk with them in their presence, the format is designed to sensitize workers to potential positive and negative effects of common professional ways of speaking. Many participants have found this process very helpful. They have described it as useful in listening in the role of the "family voice" and in receiving feedback from the person in that role. Feedback from the "family voice" has been direct, sometimes confrontational, and often quite profound for participants. The power of the format grows over time. Shaheer, who institutionalized this format into his program, describes its effects.

> We use the family voice exercise in our multidisciplinary team meeting and anytime we have structured conversations about kids and families. We assign someone to listen from the perspective of a particular child or family member and then we have questions that we use to interview that person afterwards. Initially, it was a bit awkward to follow such a structured format and there was some hesitation to do it. But I really pushed people to stick with it and we've moved from a place where people would just turn to the person in the role of the "family voice," and wait for them to speak, to actively interviewing that person and that has

gone much better. And now that voice is much stronger and forceful. For example, recently there was an exchange between a direct care counselor and our psychiatrist. So there are age differences, power differentials, and all these things that are in the room, right? And this counselor who was listening from the perspective of the kid just, straight up, gave some really direct feedback to the psychiatrist. And it was spot on. The counselor, listening from the kid's perspective, said, "That really kind of hurt when you said XYZ and I really didn't appreciate it." And the psychiatrist heard the feedback and she took it in and we moved on and it was almost like nobody even thought twice about it, but I was amazed. That would not have happened 6 months ago.

And what other effects has that format had on helpers' work?

I think it just gets us back focused on why we're all here. Sometimes we get lost in all the muck of our work and this format helps reconnect us to the work we're doing with the family. Because without the kid and family, none of us have jobs. I mean that's really what this is all about. So it helps us focus and hone in on that and it keeps us honest.

The "family voice" format has become one of the most powerful organizational interventions we have come across. The power of the "family voice" grows over time and it holds great potential to help hold workers and agencies to the ABCs of this practice (accountability, believing in possibilities, and collaboration). At the same time, there are some important considerations we want to highlight in the use of this process. It is important that participants fully agree to participate and authorize the "family voice" to give them candid feedback. It's also important that team members who are discussing a family have permission to be inadvertently offensive in their comments as long as they are willing to receive feedback about and address the effects of those comments. It helps when there is a foundation of trust in the group. At times, the person in the "family voice" role has spoken bluntly and passionately, and this process works best when it is done lovingly and in a way that honors workers' best intentions. One danger of this process is that it can have silencing effects on workers who may respond by only saying "nice, positive" things about families. The intention in this process is not to sanitize our conversations about families but to help workers increase their sensitivity to the effects of unexamined professional ways of talking and to find respectful ways of having difficult conversations about family members.

There are times when the "family voice" might be less useful; for example, when a helper wants to examine difficult personal reactions to family members, and the conversation is more focused on the helper than the family. In those times, it's important to be clear about the purpose of the conversation. If the conversation is focused on a helper's own emotional responses to a particular problem that helper should be able to define who should be included in the consultation. If a family is being discussed, the inclusion of their voice is paramount. We recognize this is a slippery slope but would suggest that if we are unclear, we act in a way that takes greater care of people's voices because they are the ones who are most at risk for becoming marginalized. Finally, the process has raised interesting questions about who to include as the "family voice." Generally, groups have found it useful to pick a perspective they would find interesting or to seek out the most marginalized voice in a particular situation. Often this voice is not a family member. Some of the more interesting "voices" have been those of other helpers. We've also found that this process can be very useful in management discussions about "difficult" employees.

BUILDING ORGANIZATIONAL CULTURES THAT SUPPORT COLLABORATION

Home-based, community-centered work often occurs against a backdrop of urgency, blame, and defensive practice (or what frontline workers more often call CYA or "covering your butt"). While this is particularly true in Child Protective Services, it can also apply across other contexts. Let's begin with urgency. As a reader, how many coworkers do you know who would say the pace of this work has slowed down and become easier over the course of their careers? Too often, helping workers operate with fewer resources and increased demands for administrative and financial accountability. In a survey of 2,200 social care professionals in England, over half said that they spent more than 60% of their time on administrative work as opposed to direct contact with people served, while more than one fifth spent over 80% of their time on such tasks, and 95% felt "that social work had become more bureaucratic and less client-focused over the previous 5 years" (Samuel, 2005, p. 8).

That was a number of years ago and many frontline workers would contend that things have slid downhill since then. A commitment to direct contact with the people we serve increasingly competes with the real demands of the bureaucratic tasks of case management. This sense of urgency and crisis is driven by the systemic shift toward data collection—the completion of forms and checklists as the primary measures of quality improvement. The impact on workers is a pervasive feeling of incompetence, a loss of meaning and conviction, and a growing belief that the work is simply not feasible.

This sense of urgency is often exacerbated by a persistent culture of blame throughout the health and human service industries. Families can feel blamed by workers for their lack of progress, workers can feel blamed by supervisors for their lack of progress, supervisors can feel blamed by administrators for incomplete attainment of organizational goals, and administrators can feel blamed by the public, the media, and the government for not preventing human tragedies that Eileen Munro (2004, p. 1090) has described as "too imperfectly understood to be predicted and prevented with certainty." In this context, there is increased questioning of worker judgment and calls for accountability. While this is completely understandable in the face of a broader professional culture that has historically clung tightly to a "leave us alone and let us do our job" ethos, we fear that in our attempts to develop services that are rightfully accountable to funders, we have moved from "measuring what is valuable" to "valuing what is measurable" (Madsen, 2007a).

The combined effects of urgency and blame have had devastating effects on both workers and the organizations that employ them. A study of why helping workers leave their jobs quoted by Eileen Munro (2004) highlights six primary reasons why workers leave, all of which can be linked in some ways to broader changes the entire field has encountered in recent years:

1. The sense of being overwhelmed by bureaucracy, paperwork, and targets
2. Insufficient resources, leading to unmanageable workloads
3. A lack of autonomy
4. Feeling undervalued by government, managers, and the public
5. Pay that is not felt to be fair
6. A change agenda that feels imposed and irrelevant

At the same time that workers are feeling less supported, agencies find themselves in an increasingly litigious environment. In that context, they become justifiably concerned about liability and the potential for lawsuits. One strategy for reducing this risk is to engage in what Eileen Munro (2004, p. 1090) refers to as "protocolization." She describes this as

> Introducing more and more formal procedures to guide practices so that they create a "correct" way to deal with a case. Then if a tragedy occurs, the agency can claim the defense of "due diligence" and show that their employees followed the correct procedures (although they did not lead to the correct outcome in terms of averting the tragedy). The success of this defensive strategy can be seen in child protection where the inquiry into the death of a child by carers concentrates more on whether the procedures were properly followed than whether the professionals made accurate assessments or decisions.

This combination of urgency, blame, and defensive practice takes an incredible toll on the work. In the face of urgency, workers become tempted to take shortcuts to survive. Fearing blame, these efforts often become covert. The combination leads to a situation in which workers can often end up feeling helpless that they can't do more and worried that they are not doing enough. This can lead to increased isolation and a sense of going "underground" in the work. This creates a "lose-lose" situation that encourages liability-driven practice, similar to a metaphorical baseball game in the bottom of the 9th inning—tied game, bases loaded, and two outs with a full count. Anxiety focuses our attention on trying to avoid a strike out rather than relaxing to put the ball in play. In this troubling context, effective helping work at a frontline level requires buffering people from the insidious effects of urgency, blame, and defensive practice. While the increasing use of relationship-based approaches like Collaborative Helping help build an organizational culture of reflection, appreciation, and shared learning, these efforts are enhanced by organizational practices that foster this same spirit. Let's examine the impact of organizational climate and culture and how it is built in daily interactions. Then we'll explore concrete ways to further embed a collaborative spirit in the tapestry of organizational climate and culture.

Charles Glisson and colleagues have done extensive research about the influence of organizational climate and culture on our work. In one study of 250 children served by 32 public children's service offices in Tennessee, they found that a strong organizational climate, characterized by low conflict, high cooperation, role clarity, and strong workplace relationships, was the primary predictor of positive service outcomes and a significant predictor of service quality (Glisson & Hemmelgarn, 1998). In another nationwide study of mental health clinics in 26 different states, they found that agencies with healthy, strong organizational climates had *half* the employee turnover and sustained new programs for *twice* as long as other organizations (Glisson et al., 2008). The stronger organizational climates were characterized by high expectations of workers who had input into management decisions, had discretion and flexibility to do their work, and were encouraged to seek out new and innovative ways of working. Workers had a clear sense of how they fit in the organization, a sense of support in their work, and buffers against work overload and emotional exhaustion. Interestingly, this coincides with research on organizational resilience that suggests the importance of emotional support for workers, high expectations of them coupled with a belief in worker success, opportunities for workers to contribute, and an organizational tolerance for ambiguity and change (Sheridan, 2012).[2] The combination of these studies highlights the importance of organizational climate at a number of levels. There are benefits for both people served and helping workers. In addition, there are powerful bottom line financial implications. The cost of replacing workers has been estimated at 40% to 70% of their annual salary, when all related costs of recruiting, hiring, retraining, and team and organizational disruption factors are considered. Improving organizational culture in service organizations not only creates the possibility of better helping, it turns out to be good business as well.

Organizational climate and culture are created daily through interactions. How people in an organization interact is profoundly influenced by the organizational culture. At the same time, those interactions shape the organizational culture. Understanding this, we can begin to identify leadership practices that help to bring a spirit of reflection, appreciation, and shared learning into the tapestry of an organizational culture. Let's begin by tracing out how two different leaders have adapted their own leadership styles to help shift organizational culture. Here is Shaheer again talking about some of the difficulties of building a family-centered residential program and his responses to those challenges.

The reality of our work is that we are very under-resourced. I have tried hard to raise the bar and insist that we're not going to do the easy thing; we're going to do the right thing. But, sometimes that's more time intensive and because we have such a dearth of resources, we at times have developed some bad habits and shortcuts to deal with the overload. And I think residential treatment historically has had some philosophical ideas about parents that are quite entrenched, especially for staff who've been here a long time. I think they can see parents as failures on some level and that's tough to break.

I think that's a pretty common experience for programs that are trying to become more family-centered. How have you dealt with that?

I try to be really clear on where we're headed and why, and when people do stuff that runs counter to that, I call them on it and I try to encourage that among my administrative team.

Can you give me an example of calling people on this?

Sure, I'll say, "I noticed that you scheduled that appointment with so and so. Did you call the family about this?" And I'll hear, "Oh, no, I didn't." And I'll simply reply, "Okay, so you need to cancel the appointment." Really? Yeah, really. We're not moving forward without checking with the family first, you know that's how we do it here. And I think you've got to be consistent and convey a message that we are very serious about this.

And are there suggestions you might have for other leaders interested in developing their own version of your ABCs?

You have to practice what you preach, right? If I'm saying that we have to believe in the possibility of success for every kid and family, then I also need to believe that the workers in this program are here because they genuinely want to help kids and families. Maybe their way of going about it is at odds with mine, but I've got to find out what their intentions are and respect what they bring.

In another realm, Anthony is the director of a number of well-established wraparound programs. When asked what he is most proud of in the development of these programs, he responds,

I think it has something to do with removing the judgmental aspect of working with families and helping our workers treat the folks they're working with more like regular people. We are not a therapy program, but all human service programs seem to have been influenced by what we might refer to as "therapy culture," which traditionally has focused on unconscious motives. I think that emphasis on interpreting "what is really going on for people" creates barriers between helpers and the people we work with and creates a very uncomfortable situation for them. We have put considerable energy into helping people examine such assumptions.

We can approach someone with a preconceived notion that we have to find out what is "really going on," or we can listen to them closely, take them at their word, and appreciate what we hear as their truth at this point in time. It may change later, but this is what it is right now. It doesn't mean we have to agree with everything they tell us. This can be a powerfully engaging experience for the people we serve. I believe we need to move beyond this idea of over-emphasizing professional expertise and really try to honor both our own knowledge and that of the people we work with.

And how have you built organizational cultures that support that belief?

If I want staff to take seriously the idea that it is okay to listen and take what people are saying at face value, then our administrative team has to do the same with staff. Much of my work over the last 15 years has been developing pilot programs where we are attempting to implement a particular model, and there is often a lot of emphasis on model fidelity and making sure that people are doing the model correctly. And that can be problematic. You can't say to staff, "Here is the right way to do it" and then get frustrated when they don't do it correctly right away. I've come to believe the best approach is a developmental one that appreciates where staff is right now and focuses on what is the one or two next steps for them towards better practice. In order to do that you have to listen to them and learn their understanding of a model, how they are implementing it, and what support they think they need to be better. When we listen for their truth, rather than ours, people are more motivated to do the work. That holds true for both families and staff.

We try to create programs that "grow staff." I like the metaphor of a garden. Gardens test your patience. You can't buy a rose bush, plant it and have perfectly formed blossoms immediately.

You have to nurture it along, and that requires water and sun-
light and attention. You need to be able to tolerate the fact that
people are going to take time to develop and try to focus on their
growth rather than the areas where they're falling short. Otherwise
you lose people.

To stay with a gardening metaphor, it seems important to create an environment within the program where people can grow.
So I guess then the question becomes what are the necessary
conditions for growth? Off the top of my head, I would say that
folks need to be inspired. They need consistent structure, limits,
and expectations. They need to feel safe to make mistakes or talk
about their mistakes or areas where they do not feel confident.
They need ways to get better and procedures in place to track,
recognize, and acknowledge small signs of progress and growth.
They need encouragement. And, they need to feel that all the
hard work is appreciated and recognized.

Both these leaders have described efforts to shift organizational culture through how they interact with frontline workers and to do that in
ways that conveyed to workers that they "matter." Andrew Turnell
(2010, p. 39), a consultant who has been instrumental in the development of signs of safety, a solution-focused approach to child protective
work, echoes the importance of these efforts in his own experiences of
trying to organizationally support implementation of signs of safety.

A collaborative, strengths-based practice approach that demands
rigorous thinking, emotional intelligence and compassion will be
undermined in an organizational culture that privileges audit
compliance and command and control leadership. I have seen
time and again that when an agency's CEO and senior management have a deep acuity to the realities of frontline practice and
a strong connection to their field staff this always creates a deeper
and more sustained implementation of Signs of Safety. Conversely,
where senior management take and/or communicate the attitude
that direct practice and practice theory and frameworks are something for practitioners, supervisors and perhaps middle management to deal with, the organizational ground for growing depth
of practice is significantly less fertile.

We think this holds true for implementation of any collaborative,
strengths-based practice framework. It is even truer for the sustainability
of any genuine helping effort. With this in mind, let's examine one

organizational practice that can bring forward reflection, appreciation, and shared learning.

Use of Appreciative Inquiry with Work Teams

Throughout this book, we have highlighted stories of good practice from both helpers and people served. The stories from workers were often collected through questions such as "What for you is at the heart of good helping? Can you tell us a story about how you put that into practice? What did you do? What challenges did you encounter? How did you respond to those challenges? What might be lessons from those experiences for our field?" This is an example of practice-based evidence, of growing practice from the ground up based on workers' everyday best moments. While this process (based more or less on the same areas of inquiry as the Collaborative Helping maps) yielded rich material for this book, it also had profound effects on the workers and teams involved in them. For example, Lindsay, a home-based worker in Chapter 2, offered a description of her work as a "thought explorer"— someone who asks questions to help people explore their thoughts in a way that creates space for them to look at their situation and have a different experience of themselves in the process. We find "thought exploring" a wonderful description of the process of inquiry and are grateful to her for allowing us to include it in this book. At the same time, Lindsay struggled with ways in which she felt marginalized in her work because of a lack of credentials. In the course of the interview, she was asked what a master's program in thought exploring might consist of, what courses might be offered, what competencies students might emerge with, and what impact it might have for both workers and people seeking help if thought exploring was more a part of our field. At the end of this interview, some of her teammates offered reflections on what it was like for them to listen to this story and the ways in which they had been moved by it. Their witnessing had a powerful effect on Lindsay. This was further enhanced a week later when her teammates presented her with a set of business cards that had her name, contact information, and the job description "thought explorer" on it. Some months later, Lindsay was at a conference in which a videotape of the interview with her about thought exploring was shown (with her permission, of course), which led to further acknowledgment of her work.

Interviews such as these can be a powerful organizational intervention. In a number of agencies, we have used appreciative inquiry to collect and share "stories from the field" as a way of honoring workers' everyday best practices. This has validating and acknowledging effects on workers, builds a sense of community, and engages a team in reflecting on their work. It can contribute to an organizational culture of reflection, appreciation, and shared learning and build practice depth by engaging workers in thinking about why they are doing what they are doing.

Typically, in this process we have begun by eliciting a recent "better moment" in a helper's work. This may range from a great moment to an okay moment to a small flicker of light in a really dark situation (we are focusing on the direction rather than the magnitude of that moment). We then get concrete details about what happened, *what* they did and *how* they did it, and what they particularly appreciated about *how* they did what they did. We also ask about some of the challenges that came up for them in that moment and how they responded to those challenges in ways that they appreciated. One of the things we've found with a more standard appreciative inquiry that only focuses on best moments and practices rather than including inquiry into accompanying difficulties is that it can be experienced by workers as minimizing those challenges and encouraging them to engage in "happy talk" that can leave them feeling unheard and unacknowledged.

That experience can lead to what David Nylund and Victor Corsiglia (1994) have referred to as "solution-forced" work rather than solution-focused work in which the consultant's agenda for best moments trumps the worker's experience of challenges in that moment. We have learned from the inevitable sighs and eye-rolling that this may not be the most helpful interaction. We also think a focus on responses to challenges provides an opportunity to further deepen inquiry into best practices. Finally, we seek to learn about what makes these "better moments" important to them, the meaning that holds for them, and what lessons there might be for the team from that moment. Afterward, we typically take some reflections from other team members where they are invited to share some of the ways in which they were moved in listening to the story and what they might want to carry back into their own work from that story.

This format has also been incorporated as a regular part of team meetings or group supervisions in which a team leader would solicit a volunteer for a brief 15-minute "best moment" interview; asking about the concrete details of those best moments, challenges and responses, and potential lessons for the team. Dan, a senior manager in an innovative child welfare department, has described the weekly use of these 15-minute interviews as one of the most powerful organizational interventions he has encountered. From his account, it has helped to shift their team culture toward a focus on possibilities and resourcefulness, an appreciation for the respective contributions of different team members, a collaborative sense of shared learning on the team, and a momentary slowing down amid the everyday frenzy of the work. As he put it,

> People walk out of the room feeling taller than when they walked in. That has also spread to other aspects of our work where we're often drawing out good work and spreading it in our everyday conversations. So now, we're more aware of thinking about what is working here and where else might it work.

This emphasis on "what's working and how we can build on that" has also rippled out in their work with children and families.

A Brief Look Back

As we said at the beginning, this book is about helping people. We have tried to cast a wide net and write something that would be accessible and applicable to a broad range of both formal and informal helpers. One hope we have had for this book is to expand how our field thinks about the process of helping and to do so in a way that acknowledges, validates, and legitimizes the daily efforts of frontline practitioners. Talking with many creative and committed helpers in the course of writing this book has been a gift for us and has touched us deeply. We also hope that this book brings forward the importance of the attitude with which helpers approach individuals, families, and communities. The people we serve deserve respect, seek connection, can best be met with curiosity, and are bolstered by hope for a better day. If our work reflects this spirit, both workers and the people we intend to help are more likely to thrive.

Collaborative Helping is a broad principle-based framework with durable cornerstones of engaging in "disciplined improvisation," realizing the core importance of relational connection, working with the life stories that make up people's sense of identity, and thoughtful questioning that supports a shift from perceived expert to genuine ally.

Collaborative Helping maps are a central feature of this practice framework. We have examined multiple ways in which they have been used across many different settings, including outreach and home-based supportive services, child protection, residential care, and even community-centered health care. The maps guide inquiry into the four areas of Vision (Where do you hope to be headed in your life?), Obstacles (What gets in the way of that Vision?), Supports (What contributes to that Vision?) and Plan (How can we draw on Supports to address Obstacles to help you move in the direction of your Vision?). This structure assists workers to focus their own thinking in uncertain, ambiguous, and complicated situations and bring some internal structure to the everyday messiness of this work. The maps also offer an organized framework for engaging people in conversations about difficult issues in their lives. Many workers have reported that having such a structure in mind keeps the conversation focused without being overly restrictive and provides a way to transparently set out on a joint venture with individuals and families. We've also found that use of these maps over time promotes powerful shifts in helping relationships. At times workers have approached us and asked, "Do you have any ideas on how I can get better in this work?" In the past, if we were not thinking it through, we might have quipped, "Yes, ground your work in a relational stance of an appreciative ally and a spirit of respect, connection, curiosity, and hope." But that encouragement is too big and vague to fully embrace. We've found that the use of the maps over time often has the same result. The maps, when used to guide conversations, shift how workers position themselves with the people they serve.

These maps provide a concrete way to help workers put the following commitments into practice:

- Striving for cultural curiosity and honoring family wisdom
- Believing in possibilities and eliciting resourcefulness
- Working in partnership and on family turf
- Engaging in empowering processes and making our work accountable to those we serve

In this way, these maps support a culturally responsive, strengths-based, collaborative, and accountable practice.

We moved from the broad use of Collaborative Helping maps to guide our work to a more detailed consideration of the processes of engagement, visioning, and talking about obstacles and supports. We began with the question of how we can connect with people to help them reflect on their hopes and visions for their lives. There is an interesting interplay here between relational connection and visioning. People's willingness to enter into a conversation about their hopes and purposes in life requires the establishment of trust, and conversations about vision, hopes, and purposes contribute to meaningful relationships. Realizing that these efforts can be difficult at times, we outlined concrete suggestions on ways to engage reluctant individuals and families and develop vision in situations awash in crisis or hopelessness. We also emphasized that the process of eliciting vision is more complicated than simply asking, "What's your vision for your life?" With that in mind, we offered a variety of concrete ways to build a bridge that helps people step into these conversations and feel attended to in the process.

We continued our exploration of the intricacies of the work with a focus on ways of talking about obstacles and supports. We took up the unusual and creative use of externalizing from narrative approaches to view people and problems as separate entities that are in a changeable relationship with each other. This is a shift from "I am stuck with the fact that I have a problem or I am a problem" to "I am in a relationship with this problem that has come into my life and I bet I can change that relationship." This shift in thinking enhances people's sense of influence and participation in their own lives and opens up more options for responding to problems. Likewise, we explored some different ways of conceptualizing strengths and supports. Rather than considering strengths as internal personality characteristics ("I am a respectful person"), we highlighted ways to view strengths as practices in life ("How do you *do* respect in your life? How do you put respect into practice?"). We then examined ways that such practices might be linked to people's broader intentions, values and beliefs, hopes and dreams, and commitments in life, and further supported by important others in their lives. These newer ways of thinking about problems and strengths, in and of themselves, can powerfully shift helping work. To take that further, we also outlined concrete guidelines for actual conversations with people about problems and strengths that flow out of this approach and gave numerous examples of some resulting exchanges.

We have repeatedly sought to view home and community work through a lens of "walking and talking"—a creative mix of concrete assistance coupled with thoughtful conversation that can make our work both immediately relevant and transformative. Home and community work offers many opportunities for innovative work. There are also numerous challenges and dilemmas, and we shared a number of stories about creative responses to some of those dilemmas. And finally, we laid out some ideas at supervisory and organizational levels to support collaborative ways of working and embed these ideas and practices in the fabric of organizational culture. The use of Collaborative Helping maps at supervisory and organizational levels institutionalizes a shift from corrective instruction to facilitative inquiry. Overall, the incorporation of these ideas and practices at multiple levels (frontline practice, supervision, and organizational functioning) builds and sustains a context that supports a collaborative spirit.

By way of closing, we want to emphasize that this book has been an attempt to bring together learned and lived knowledge. We trust that our ideas about Collaborative Helping will provide a useful framework that helps to organize your own thought process as well as the conversations you have with people as you help them with the everyday tasks of life. We also hope that the framework encourages a celebration of the wisdom gained from your own experience of doing your work. This book has grown from the ground up through the everyday experience of frontline practitioners and the people they serve. Wisdom about effective helping comes as much from the lived experience of individuals, families, communities, and workers as it does from more traditional empirically based evidence. As we have said before, both are important and work best together in a holistic fashion. While we believe this framework will be useful and encourage you to adapt it to a best fit for you in your everyday work, we also hope our description of Collaborative Helping validates your sense of what is important in this work and encourages you to continue to learn from your own lived experience. Accept our best wishes for an exciting and rewarding journey.

NOTES

1. The inclusion of questions about purpose, context, and stakeholders in this map draws from a dialogue structure for supervision and consultation developed by John Vogel and Sophia Chin of the Massachusetts Child Welfare Institute, the child protective services training arm in that state. Bill is indebted to them for extensive conversations and inspiration in our shared work.

2. You'll note that we made a similar connection in Chapter 7 in relation to resilience with people, families, and communities.

References

Benard, B. (2004). *Resiliency: What we have learned.* San Francisco, CA: WestEd.

Benard, B. (2006). Using strengths-based practice to tap the resilience of families. In D. Saleebey (Ed.), *The strengths perspective in social work practice* (4th ed.). Boston, MA: Pearson.

Berg, I. K. (1991). Of visitors, complainants, and customers: Is there really such a thing as resistance? *Family Therapy Networker, 13*, 21.

Berg, I. K. (1994). *Family based services: A solution-focused approach.* New York, NY: W.W. Norton.

Berg, I. K. & Kelly, S. (2000). *Building solutions in child protective services.* New York, NY: Norton.

Berg, I. K. & Miller, S. D. (1992). *Working with the problem drinker: A solution-focused approach.* New York, NY: Norton.

Blue-Banning, M., Summers, J. A., Nelson, L. L., Frankland, C., & Beegle, G. P. (2004). Dimensions of family and professional partnerships: Constructive guidelines for collaboration. *Exceptional Children, 70*(2), 167–184.

Boyd-Franklin, N. (1989). *Black families in clinical practice.* New York, NY: Jason Aronson.

Boyd-Franklin, N., & Bry, N. H. (2000). *Reaching out in family therapy: Home-based, school, and community interventions.* New York, NY: Guilford Press.

Bruns, E. J., & Walker, J. S. (2008). Ten principles of the wraparound process. In E. J. Bruns & J. S. Walker (Eds.), *The resource guide to wraparound.* Portland, OR: National Wraparound Initiative, Research and Training Center for Family Support and Children's Mental Health.

Burchard, J. D., Bruns, E. J., & Burchard, S. N. (2002). The wraparound approach. In B. Burns & K. Hoagwood (Eds.), *Community treatment for youth: Evidence-based interventions for severe emotional and behavioral disorders* (pp. 69–90). New York, NY: Oxford University Press.

Bureau of Labor Statistics, U.S. Department of Labor. (2012–2013). *Occupational outlook handbook.* Retrieved 10/1/13 from http://www.bls.gov/ooh/

Butterworth, P. (2000). Talking about self-care in relation to using drugs. *Gecko: A Journal of Deconstruction and Narrative Ideas in Therapeutic Practice, 3*, 64–76.

Crowe, T. (2006). *Some externalising questions in relation to addictive thinking (self).* Retrieved 4/30/06 from www.dulwichcentre.com.au

Christensen, D. N., Todahl, J., & Barrett, W. C. (1999). *Solution-based casework: An introduction to clinical and case management skills in casework practice.* London, England: Aldine Transaction.

Cooperrider, D. L. (2000). Positive image, positive action: The affirmative basis of organiz-ing. In D. L. Cooperrider, P. F. Sorensen, D. Whitney, & T. F. Yaeger (Eds.), *Appreciative inquiry: Rethinking human organization toward a positive theory of change* (pp. 29–54). Champaign, IL: Stipes Publishing.

Cooperrider, D. L., Sorensen, P. F., Whitney, D., & Yaeger, T. F. (Eds.). (2000). *Appreciative inquiry: Rethinking human organization toward a positive theory of change.* Champaign, IL: Stipes Publishing.

Cooperrider, D. L., Whitney, D., & Stavros, J. M. (2008). *Appreciative inquiry handbook* (2nd ed.). Brunswick, OH: Crown Custom Publishing.

Dennis, K. W., & Lourie, I. S. (2006). *Everything is normal until proven otherwise: A book about wraparound services.* Washington, DC: Child Welfare League of America.

de Shazer, S. (1985). *Keys to solution in brief therapy.* New York, NY: Norton.

de Shazer, S. (1988). *Clues: Investigating solutions in brief therapy.* New York, NY: Norton.

Dickerson, V. C. (2010). Positioning oneself within an epistemology: Refining our thinking about integrative approaches. *Family Process, 49*(3), 349–368.

Duncan, B. L., Miller, S. D., & Sparks, J. (2004). *The heroic client: A revolutionary way to improve effectiveness through client-directed, outcome-informed therapy* (Rev. ed.). San Francisco, CA: Jossey-Bass.

Duncan, B. L., Miller, S. D., Sparks, J., Claud, D., Reynolds, L., Brown, J., & Johnson, L. (2003). The session rating scale: Preliminary psychometric properties of a working alli-ance measure. *Journal of Brief Therapy, 3*, 3–12.

Duncan, B. L., Miller, S. D., Wambold B. E., & Hubble, M. A. (2010). *The heart and soul of change* (2nd ed.). Washington, DC: American Psychological Association.

Durrant, M. (1993). *Residential treatment: A cooperative, competency-based approach to therapy and program design.* New York, NY: Norton.

Freedman, J., & Combs, G. (1996). *Narrative therapy: The social construction of preferred realities.* New York, NY: Norton.

Freeman, J. C., Epston, D., & Lobovits, D. H. (1997). *Playful approaches to serious problems: Narrative therapy with children and their families.* New York, NY: Norton.

Freire, P. (1981). *Pedagogy of the oppressed.* New York, NY: Continuum Publishing.

Gehart, D. R. (2012a). The mental health recovery movement and family therapy, Part I: Consumer-led reform of services to persons diagnosed with severe mental illness. *Journal of Marital and Family Therapy, 38*(3), 429–442.

Gehart, D. R. (2012b). The mental health recovery movement and family therapy, Part II: A collaborative, appreciative approach to supporting mental health recovery. *Journal of Marital and Family Therapy, 38*(3), 443–457.

Glisson, C., & Hemmelgarn, A. L. (1998). The effects of organizational climate and inter-organizational coordination on the quality and outcomes of children's service systems. *Child Abuse and Neglect, 22*(5), 401–421.

Glisson, C., Schoenwald, S. K., Kelleher, K., Landsverk, J., Hoagwood, K. E., Mayberg, S., & Green, P. (2008). Therapist turnover and new program sustainability in mental health clinics as a function of organizational culture, climate, and service structure. *Administration and Policy in Mental Health and Mental Health Services Research, 35*(1), 124–133.

Hammond, S. A. (1998). *The thin book of appreciative inquiry* (2nd ed.). Plano, TX: Thin Book Publishing.

Heath, C., & Heath, D. (2007). *Made to stick: Why some ideas survive and others die*. New York, NY: Random House.

Henggeler, S. W., Cunningham, P. B., Schoenwald, S. K., & Borduin, C. M. (2009). *Multisystemic therapy for antisocial behavior in children and adolescents*. New York, NY: Guilford Press.

Jenkins, A. (1990). *Invitations to responsibility: The therapeutic engagement of men who are violent and abusive*. Adelaide, Australia: Dulwich Centre Publication.

Kegan, R., & Laskow Lahey, L. (2000). *How the way we talk can change the way we work: Seven languages for transformation*. San Francisco, CA: Jossey-Bass.

Kliman, J., & Trimble, D. (1983). Network therapy. In B. Wolman & G. Stricker (Eds.), *Handbook of family and marital therapy* (pp. 277–314). New York, NY: Plenum.

Madigan, S. (2010). *Narrative therapy*. Washington, DC: APA Press.

Madsen, W. C. (1992). Problematic treatment: Interaction of patient, spouse and physician beliefs in medical noncompliance. *Family Systems Medicine, 10*(4), 365–383.

Madsen, W. C. (1996). Integrating a "client voice" in clinical training. *American Family Therapy Academy Newsletter, 64*, 24–26.

Madsen, W. C. (1999). *Collaborative therapy with multi-stressed families: From old problems to new futures*. New York, NY: Guilford Press.

Madsen, W. C. (2004). Sustaining a collaborative clinical practice in the "real" world. In S. Madigan (Ed.), *Therapy from the outside in*. Vancouver, BC: Yaletown Family Therapy.

Madsen, W. C. (2006). Teaching across discourses to sustain collaborative clinical practice. *Journal of Systemic Therapies, 25*(4), 44–58.

Madsen, W. C. (2007a). *Collaborative therapy with multi-stressed families* (2nd ed.). New York, NY: Guilford Press.

Madsen, W. C. (2007b). Working within traditional structures to support a collaborative clinical practice. *The International Journal of Narrative Therapy and Community Work, 2*, 51–62.

Madsen, W. C. (2009). Collaborative helping: A practice framework for family-centered services. *Family Process, 48*, 103–116.

Madsen, W. C. (2011). Collaborative helping maps: A tool to guide thinking and action in family-centered services. *Family Process, 50*, 529–543.

Man-kwong, H. (2004). Overcoming craving: The use of narrative practices in breaking drug habits. *The International Journal of Narrative Therapy and Community Work, 1*, 17–24.

Meyerhoff, B. (1982). Life history among the elderly: Performance, visibility and re-membering. In J. Ruby (Ed.), *A crack in the mirror: Reflexive perspectives in anthropology*. Philadelphia, PA: University of Pennsylvania Press.

Meyerhoff, B. (1986). Life not death in Venice: Its second life. In V. W. Turner & E. M. Bruner (Eds.), *The anthropology of experience* (pp. 261–286). Chicago, IL: University of Illinois Press.

Miller, B. F., Kessler, R., Peek, C. J., & Kallenberg, G. A. (2011, July). A national agenda for research in collaborative care: Papers from the collaborative care research network research development conference. *AHRQ Publication No. 11-0067*. Rockville MD: Agency for Healthcare Research and Quality.

Miller, S., Duncan, B., Brown, J., Sparks, J., & Claud, D. (2003). The outcome rating scale: A preliminary study of reliability, validity, and feasibility of a brief visual analog measure. *Journal of Brief Therapy, 2*, 91–100.

Miller, W. R., & Rollnick, S. (2002). *Motivational interviewing: Preparing people for change* (2nd ed). New York, NY: Guilford.

Miller, W. R., & Rollnick, S. (2013). *Motivational interviewing: Helping people change* (3rd ed). New York, NY: Guilford.

Monk, G., Winslade, J., Crocket, K., & Epston, D. (Eds.). (1997). *Narrative therapy in practice: The archaeology of hope.* San Francisco, CA: Jossey-Bass.

Morgan, A. (2000). *What is narrative therapy? An easy-to-read introduction.* Adelaide, Australia: Dulwich Centre Press.

Munro, E. (2004). The impact of audit on social work practice. *British Journal of Social Work, 36,* 1075–1095.

Nylund, D., & Corsiglia, V. (1994). Becoming solution-focused forced in brief therapy: Remembering something important we already knew. *Journal of Systemic Therapies, 13*(1), 5–12.

Parker, S. (2013). The future house tool: Involving parents and caregivers in the safety planning process. Retrieved 10/2/2013 from www.spconsultancy.com.au

Parker, S. (in preparation). *The safety planning tool.* Distributed by author. It will be available at www.spconsultancy.com.au

Parton, N., & O'Byrne, P. (2000). *Constructive social work: Towards a new practice.* London, England: MacMillan Press.

Pulleyblank Coffey, E. (2004). The heart of the matter 2: Integration of ecosystemic family therapy practices with systems of care mental health services for children and families. *Family Process, 43,* 161–174.

Root, E. A., & Madsen, W. C. (2013). Imagine: Bringing vision into child protective services. *Journal of Systemic Therapies, 32*(3), 76–91.

Rothstein, D., & Santana, L. (2011). *Make just one change: Teach students to ask their own questions.* Cambridge, MA: Harvard Education Press.

Russell, S., & Carey, M. (2004). *Narrative therapy: Responding to your questions.* Adelaide, Australia: Dulwich Centre Publications.

Samuel, M. (2005). Social care professionals overwhelmed by paperwork. *Community Care, 14,* 8.

Sheinberg, M., & Fraenkel, P. (2001). *The relational trauma of incest: A family-based approach to treatment.* New York, NY: Guilford Press.

Sheridan, K. (2012). *Building a magnetic culture: How to attract and retain top talent to create an engaged, productive workforce.* New York, NY: McGraw Hill.

Sobell, L. (2013, June 13). *Using motivational interviewing with difficult clients.* Keynote address at International Social Work Conference sponsored by University of Applied Sciences Northwestern Switzerland. Olten, Switzerland.

Tomm, K. (1987a). Interventive interviewing: Part I. Strategizing as a fourth guideline for the therapist. *Family Process, 26,* 3–13.

Tomm, K. (1987b). Interventive interviewing: Part II. Reflexive questioning as a means to enable self-healing. *Family Process, 26,* 167–183.

Tomm, K. (1988). Interventive interviewing: Part III. Intending to ask lineal, circular, strategic or reflexive questions. *Family Process, 27,* 1–15.

Tomm, K. (1989). Externalizing the problem and internalizing personal agency. *Journal of Strategic and Systemic Therapies, 8*(1), 54–59.

Tomm, K. (1991). Beginnings of a "HIPs and PIPs" approach to psychiatric assessment. *Calgary Participator*, 21–24.

Turnell, A. (2008, March 20–21). *Signs of safety: An innovative approach to child protection work.* Workshop presented at the Family Institute of Cambridge, Watertown, MA.

Turnell, A. (2010). *The signs of safety: A comprehensive briefing paper.* Retrieved 4/22/11 from http://www.signsofsafety.net

Turnell, A., & Edwards, S. (1999). *Signs of safety: A solution and safety oriented approach to child protection casework.* New York, NY: Norton.

Turnell, A., & Essex, S. (2006). *Working with 'denied' child abuse: The resolutions approach.* New York, NY: Open University Press.

Turnell, A., & Parker, S. (2010). *The signs of safety approach: Mapping cases using the signs of safety assessment and planning framework.* Retrieved from http://www.aspirationsconsultancy.com

U.S. Department of Health and Human Services. (2004). *National consensus statement on mental recovery.* Retrieved 8/26/08 from http://menntalhealth.samhsa.gov/publications/allpubs/sma05-4129

VanDenBerg, J., Bruns, E., & Burchard, J. (2003). History of the wraparound process. *Focal Point: A National Bulletin on Family Support and Children's Mental Health, 17,* 4–7.

Walnum, E. (2007). Sharing stories: The work of an experience consultant. *The International Journal of Narrative Therapy and Community Work, 2,* 3–9.

Walsh, F. (2010). *Spiritual resources in family therapy* (2nd ed.). New York, NY: Guilford Press.

Walsh, J. (1999). *Clinical case management with persons having mental illness: A relationship-based perspective.* Boston, MA: Cengage Learning.

Webster's Third New International Dictionary. (2002). Springfield, MA: Meagan & Webster.

White, M. (1995). *Re-authoring lives: Interviews and essays.* Adelaide, Australia: Dulwich Centre Publications.

White, M. (2000). Reflections on narrative practice: Essays and interviews. Adelaide, Australia: Dulwich Centre Publications.

White, M. (2007). *Maps of narrative practice.* New York, NY: Norton.

White, M., & Epston, D. (1990). *Narrative means to therapeutic ends.* New York, NY: Norton.

Zimmerman, J. L., & Dickerson, V. C. (1996). *If problems talked: Narrative therapy in action.* New York, NY: Guilford Press.

INDEX

Page numbers in *italic* type indicate figures.

ABCs approach, 183–86, 194
accountability, 166, 173–75
  decision components, 173–74
  of helping worker, 31–33, 200
  program goals, 186–87
action plan. *See* plan
actions-intentions gap, 114
adaptation improvement,18, 101
adjectives,, switching to nouns from,
    128–30, 143
adolescent cultural beliefs, 62, 63, *67*
advice, limited effectiveness of, 40
advocacy efforts, 152, 166–75
  family partners and, 161–62
  helping workers and, 173–74
agency, 63, 148, 162
alcohol abuse, 24, 91, 93, 95, 133, 134,
    156–57
Amanda's story, 6–8, 9, 11, 13, 14, 152
Amira's story, 4–5, 9, 10, 13–14
anger, 74, 75
Angry Feelings, 74–75
anxiety, 119, 130–31
appreciative inquiry, 17, 104–5
  description of, 104
  work teams and, 197–99
asking questions. *See* questions
Asperger's syndrome, 57
assessment, 10, 11, 185
attitude. *See* relational stance

Beach Center Family-Professional
    Partnership Scale, 187
bearing witness, 11, 38
Beegle, G. P., 187

behavior
  externalizing conversations about,
    132–33
  goals and, 55, 108
  off-putting, 60
  out-of-control, 52
  sequences of, 19
behavioral health, 20–21
behavioral intervention, 19–20
belief in self, 7–8
beliefs, 142, 143, 149, 201
  cultural, 61–62, *67*
Benard, B., 155
Berg, I. K., 17, 56, 102, 108
"best moments" focus, 104–5
blame and shame
  minimizing of, 97, 125, 127, 148
  organizational culture of, 191, 192
  parenting and, 76, 101
  reduction of, 37, 59, 60–61
  self-blame and, 74–77, 1385
bleak future, 118, 119–20
Blue-Banning, M., 187
Borduin, C. M., 17–18
boundaries. *See* professional boundaries
Boyd-Franklin, N., 18
brainstorming, 75
bridge building, 13
Brown, J., 186
Bruns, E., 49
Bruns, E. J., 18
Bry, N. H., 18
Burchard, J., 49
Burchard, J. D., 18
Burchard, S. N., 18

bureaucratic pressures, 190–92
Bureau of Labor Statistics, U.S., 21
Butterworth, Paul, 145

Carey, M., 37, 127
case management, 9, 39
    meaningful conversation and, 66
    misunderstanding of, 20
    therapy vs., 8
case presentation, 178, 179
change
    growing exception into plan for, 112,
        114–15, 116, 118
    practical, 11
    questions for possibilities of, 43–46, 139
    rejection of, 109–11
    shift in focus on, 50, 170–71
Child Protective Services (CPS), 1, 2,
        11, 172
    accountability and, 31–33
    bureaucratic pressures and, 190
    Collaborative Helping maps and, 78–90
    concrete help and, 152–53
    flexible boundaries and, 155–56
    Future House visual tool and,
        106–8, 106
    parental hopes and, 55–56
    problems separated from people and,
        86–87
    signs of safety approach and, 17, 196
    supervisory consultation and, 181–83
    Vision Statement and, 80–81, 102–4
Chin, Sophia, 202n1
class, 36, 37, 58
Claud, D., 186
clinical discussion formats, 187–90
closeness, 67
codependence, 110
Collaborative Helping
    "ally" concept of, 12–13
    attitude and, 23, 199
    in broader context, 17–20
    definition of, 199
    dilemmas in, 151–75
    family partners contribution to, 159–62,
        167–73
    four cornerstones of, 46–47
    future of, 20–21

inquiry and, 23, 40–46, 50–51
life stories focus of, 1–14, 33–39, 199
organizational principles supporting,
    177–90
as principle-based approach, 23–24
relational stanceand, 23, 26–33, 115
Right Questions Project and, 174
well-established sources of, 17
See also helping workers
Collaborative Helping maps, 25–26,
    49–68, 69–98, 202
    carbon version of, 80
    Child Protective Services and, 78–90
    conversations about strengths and,
        142–44, 149
    externalizing conversations about
        problems and, 135–38, 135
    four questions and, 51
    home health care and, 91–96
    identifying obstacles and supports and,
        61–64, 62, 87
    informal version of, 91, 95, 96, 97
    organizing vision and, 67
    overview of, 50–51, 51
    plan development and, 64–67, 65, 87
    practice-based evidence and, 197
    residential programs and, 69–78
    supervision enhancement with, 177–83
    usefulness of, 68, 200
collective agency, 63
Combs, G., 127, 138
commitment, 62, 105, 143, 201
common factors literature, 26
common ground, 13
community, 105, 107
    Child Protection Services engagement
        with, 79
    development of supportive, 142, 144
    helping worker understanding of,
        119–20
    residential treatment program and,
        77–78
    resources of, 10–11, 20, 64–65
    violence and, 91
community-based work, 9, 21, 25,
    121–23, 151–75
    boundary dilemmas and, 151–75
    bureaucratic pressure and, 190

family partners and, 160–61
service hierarchy and, 162–66
supervision and, 177–83
terrain of, 153–55
See also organizational practices
compassion, 60
competence, 100, 162
complaint to commitment questions,
    104–5
concrete efforts, 10–11, 152–59, 174
concrete services. *See* case management
connection. *See* relational connection
Consiglia, Victor, 198
contact before content, 178, 180
context questions, 178
control, *67*
conversations
    collaborative, 97, 200
    effectiveness of, 127
    externalizing, 59–61, 127–39
    meaningful, 66
    open, respectful, and honest, 27
    relational connections and, 125
    about strengths, 139–49, 201
    supervisory, *179*, 180, 181
    See also walking and talking
Cooperrider, David, 17, 81, 104
coping strategies, 127
corrective-intent vs. facilitative-intent
    questions, 44–46, 139
CPS. *See* Child Protective Services
crises, perpetual, 118, 119–20, 201
Crocket, K., 127
cross-cultural negotiation, 2–4, 27–29,
    36–37, 147–48, 175. *See also*
    sociocultural context
Crowe, T., 145
cultural beliefs, 35–37, 61–62, *67*
cultural curiosity, 2–3, 27–29, 200
cultural values, 147–48, 175
Cunningham, P. B., 17–18
curiosity, 13–14, 27–29, 40, 56, 200
customer relationships, 108–9

danger scaling questions, 81
Danger Statement, 82, 83, 86–87, 88, 90
    Vision Statement and, 87
data clouds, 185

data collection, 91
decision making, 24–25
    accountable components of, 173–74
defensiveness, 59, 60, 127
definitional ceremonies, 38, 64, 118, 174
degrading rituals, 37
denial, 37–38, 108
    No Problem Stance and, 109–10,
        111, *111*
Dennis, Karl, 18, 99–100
depression, 24, 52, 58, 59, 91, 119
descriptors, 100–101
de Shazer, S., 17, 51, 102, 108
despair, 127, 132, 140–42
determination, 140–42, 143, 144
diabetes, 117, 118, 133, 140, 142
diagnostic manuals, 29, 149n3
Dickerson, V. C., 127
Dickerson, Vicki, 33
differences. *See* sociocultural context
dilemmas, 134, 151–75, 201
    in advocacy efforts, 166–75
direction, 53
disciplined improvisation, 25, 46,
    144, 199
disempowerment, 31, 161–62
documentation, 29
Doing the Vision, 84–86
    example of, 85–86
"do the right thing," 29
dreams, 142, 143, 149, 201
drugs. *See* substance misuse
Duncan, Barry, 26, 186
Durrant, Michael, 50, 71, 73

Edwards, Steve, 17, 29–30
empirical approaches, 17
empowerment, 31–33, 139, 200
enabler, 110
engagement, 99–123, 201
    proactive vision and, 102–23
    relevance and, 123
    strength-based style of, 100–101
engagement difficulties, 108–18
    little hope for future and, 120–23
    No Control Stance and, *111*, 115–18
    No Problem Stance and, 111–15
    perpetual crisis and, 118, 119–20

Epston, David, 17, 35, 59, 127
ethics, professional, 175
Everything Is Normal until Proven Otherwise (Dennis and Lourie), 18, 99–100
evidence-based practice, 17, 197
exception, 112, 114–15, 116, 118
existential problem, 95
experience, 14–17
  learned, 160, 202
  story lines and, 34–37, *34*
experiential knowledge. *See* family partners
"expert" vs. "ally" help, 12–13
extended family, 20, 65, 129, 90
externalizing, 59–63, 125, 127–39, 143, 148–49, 201
  Angry Feelings and, 74–75
  Danger Statement and, 87
  as different approach, 128
  examples of conversations, 130–34
  map for conversations, 135–38, *135*
  obstacles and, 97, 127
  own experience and, 129–30
  sociocultural context of, 138–39

facilitating-intent questions, 44, 45–46, 139
family
  changing relational pattern of, 146–47
  Child Protective Services engagement with, 79–82
  collaboratively developed plan and, 64–65
  cultural beliefs and, 61–62, *67*
  cultural "shoulds" and, 36–37
  engagement difficulties with, 108–12
  natural environment of, 36
  power dynamics with, 30–31
  residential treatment program and, 77–78, 93–94
  support from family partners and, 159–62
  Vision Statement and, 83–84, 103
  wisdom and traditions of, 27–29, 44, 52, 200
  See also extended family; home-based work

family-centered services, 49, 193–94
family partners, 159–62, 165, 167–73, 175
  challenges faced in family systems meetings, 169–70
  definition of, 159
  experiential knowledge and, 160–61, 171
  personal stories use by, 168–69
  roles of, 170, 171
family resources, 20
family safety plan, 88–91
family therapy, 19–20
family voice format, 188–90
feedback, 31, 187, 188
first do no harm, 112, 116, 117
first step, taking of, 117–18
flexibility, 58
focus
  lack of shared, 55
  on positives, 100–101, 104–5
  on possibilities, 53–54, 97, 102
forward-thinking vision, 53, 56, 125
foster care, 1, 2
Fraenkel, Peter, 101
framing problems, 73–74
Frankland, C., 187
Freedman, J., 127, 138
Freeman, J. C., 127
Freire, Paulo, 160
friends, 20, 64–65, 90
functioning, improvement in, 18, 101
future. *See* vision of life's direction
Future House (visual tool), 105–8, *106*, 123n1

gang-involved youths, 121–23, 129–30
Gehart, D. R., 101
gender, 36, 37
genuineness, 159
Glisson, Charles, 192–93
goals
  collaborative development of, 53–58
  current behavior discrepancy with, 108
  life changes and, 50–51, 53
  realistic, 56–57
  safety, 83, 88, 90
  See also vision of life's direction

Golden Rule, 32, 125
Green, P., 193
Guthrie, Woody, 33–34, 37

harm reduction program, 145
Harm Statement, 82, 83, 88, 90
    Vision Statement and, 87
health care, 20–21, 37–38
    Collaborative Helping maps and,
        91–96
    coordination of, 21
    payment system, 166
    reforms in, 18–19, 20, 49, 91, 185
    See also home health workers; medical
        conditions
hearing, 11, 12, 38
Heath, Chip and Dan, 55
Heather's story, 23–24
helping workers, 2–14, 17, 20, 46
    accountable decisions criteria and,
        173–74
    activities of, 9–12
    as ally, 12–13, 27
    appreciative inquiry and, 17, 104–5,
        197–99
    attitude of, 199
    best moments interviews and, 198, 199
    best outcomes and, 26–27
    boundary dilemmas and, 151–75
    bureaucratic stresses on, 190–92
    client relationship, 33
    Collaborative Helping maps and,
        177, 200
    commitments of, 2–3, 28–29, 38, 200
    concrete help from, 10–11, 66,
        152–53, 152–59
    core activities of, 11, 12, 38
    corrective vs. facilitative questions
        and, 139
    cost of replacing, 193
    curiosity and, 13–14, 27–29, 40,
        56, 200
    development of, 33, 45
    directness of, 4–6
    engagement and, 99–122, 201
    externalizing and, 60–66, 137–381
    family voice format and, 188–90
    habits of thought and, 177
    "in-between" state of, 24–25

inquiry and, 23, 40–46, 47, 50–51, 56,
    139–40
interactions and, 39–46, 109–10, *110*,
    118, 133–47, 156–57
marginalization of, 197
misuse of power and, 139
as nonjudgmental, 6
openness and, 3–4, 63–64
organizational culture and, 190–96
power dynamics and, 162–66
professional criticism of, 158–59
qualities of, 5, 8–9, 27
reasons for leaving job of, 191–92
relational connections building by,
    12–14, 17, 20, 46–47, 52–53, 97,
    123, 125
respect from, 27, 134
sharing own life story by, 7, 13,
    129–30, 148
showing own humanity of, 31, 154–55
simultaneous multiple realities and,
    140–41
story metaphors and, 35–37
terrain of, 153–55
themes of, 13–14
as thought explorers, 40–41, 197
traditional colleagues and, 166–75
validation by, 11
Vision Statement and, 85–86
wisdom gained by, 202
    See also community-based work;
        home-based work; home health care
Hemmelgarn, A. L., 192–93
Henggeler, S. W., 17–18
Henry's story, 1–4, 9, 10, 11, 13, 14
Hoagwood, K. E., 193
home-based work, 9, 19, 20, 21, 36, 202
    boundary dilemmas in, 151–75
    bureaucratic pressures and, 190
    Collaborative Helping maps and, 52–53
    decision making in, 24–25
    service hierarchy and, 162–66
    supervision and, 177–83
    terrain of, 153–55
    See also organizational practices
home health workers, 21, 37
    advocacy efforts and, 152, 166–75
    Collaborative Helping maps and, 91–96
    dynamics of privilege and, 163–64

homophobia, 58, 133, 134, 136, 138
hopefulness, 27
hopelessness, 75–76, 132, 201
hopes, 54, 100, 142, 143, 149, 201
  clarifying of, 178, *179*
  informal Collaborative Helping Map
    and, 92, *96*
Hubble, M. A., 26
humility, 13
hypertension, 91, 92, 93, 95, 134

identity, 14–17, 37–38, 140, 152
  as evolving, 15–16, 140–41
  as fused with problems, 127
  new stories of, 39–40
  See also self
improvisation, disciplined, 25, 46,
    144, 199
impulsivity, 39, 52, 61, *62*, 63, *67*
influence, sense of, 201
information gathering, 73–74
inner-city youth, 121–23, 129–30, 146–47
innovative care programs, 49, 202
inquiry, 23, 40–46, 47, 56, 139–40
  appreciative, 17, 104–5, 197–99
  collaborative, 50–51
  informal Collaborative Action Map
    and, 97
  See also questions
insight, 64
inspiration, 53
institutional placement, 49
instruct/resist patterns, 166–67
intentional practices
  patterns of, 149n3
  strengths of, 139–44, 148, 149, 201
intentions gap, 114
interactional patterns, 133–47
  over-responsible/under-responsible,
    133–34, *134*
  stepping out of, 146–47
invisibility, 134, 136, 138
Irsfeld, Anthony, 160–61

Kallenberg, G. A., 20
Karley's story, 42–46
Kegan, Robert, 104–5
Kelleher, K., 193
Kessler, R., 20

Landsverk, J., 193
language, accessible, 128–30, 131,
    136, 143
Laskow Lahey, Lisa, 104–5
lawsuits, state-level, 49
leadership practices, 193–94
lead from beside, 162
learned experience, 160, 202
liability-driven practice, 192
life changes
  active help toward, 11
  Collaborative Helping Map and, 51
  goals and, 50–51, 53
  organizing vision for, 53–58
  preferred direction and, 54
  sense of purpose and, 105
  See also vision of life's direction
life stories, 1–17, 23–24, 26, 46–47,
    97, 173
  bearing witness to, 11, 38
  as Collaborative Helping focus, 1–14,
    33–39, 199
  as engagement with No Problem
    Stance, 111–15
  family partners and, 168–69
  living out preferred, 66
  personal vs. private, 169
  sharing by helping worker of, 7, 13,
    129–30, 148
listening, 11
litigation, 49, 192
lived experience, 160, 202
Lobovits, D. H., 127
Lourie, Ira, 18, 99–100

macro-level innovative care programs, 49
Madsen, W. C., 13, 27, 80, 98n1, 103,
    109, 127, 138, 149n3, 166, 185, 191
Man-kwong, H., 145
maps, *See* Collaborative Helping maps
Margie s story, 16, 17
Massachusetts Child Welfare Institute,
    202n1
maximize/minimize. *See* minimize/
    maximize pattern
Mayberg, S., 193
medical conditions
  Collaborative Helping Map and, 91–96
  denial of, 37–38

determination to manage, 142
minimize/maximize sequence, *111*,
  115–16, 118, 140
See also home health care
mental health problems, 70, 110, 159
  recovery orientation, 18–19
See also depression
Merry-Go-Round, stepping off of,
  146–47
Meyerhoff, Barbara, 38
Miller, B. F., 20
Miller, Scott, 186
Miller, S. D., 26, 56, 108
Miller, W. R., 17, 108
mind the gap, 112, 113–14
minimize/maximize pattern, *111*, 115–16,
  118, 140, 166
miracle question, 102
Monk, G., 127
mood swings, 70
Morgan, A., 34–35, 127, 138
Mother Blame, 138
motivation, 107, 108
  foundation of, 105
motivational interviewing, 17, 108, 109
  four general principles, 108
multi-stressed situations, 119, 190–92
multisystemic therapy (MST), 18, 19–20
Munro, Eileen, 191, 192

Nag/Explode Thing, 61–62, *62*, *67*
narrative approaches, 38–39, 145, 149n4
  externalizing and, 59–61, 125,
    127, 201
See also life stories
narrative therapy, 34
needs rethinking, 126–27
neglect, 27, 109, 181
Nelson, L. L., 187
networks, 20, 64–65, 90, 129
network therapists, 65
No Control Stance, 109, 110–11
  engagement of woman with, *111*,
    115–18
  exceptions to, 112, 117, 118, 140, 141
  interactional patterns, 110–11, *111*
No Problem Stance, 109–10, 111
  engagement of youth with, 111–15
  interactional patterns, 109–10, *110*, 112

nouns, switching adjectives to,
  128–30, 143
Nylund, David, 198

obesity, 91, 92, 93, 95
obituary, informal, 94–95
obstacles, 51, 201
  approaches to, 54, 125
  Collaborative Helping maps and, 92,
    96, 97, *160*, *179*, 180, 200
  externalizing of, 97, 127
  identification of, 58–64, *62*, *67*, *72*,
    74, 92
  needs recast as, 126
  new ways of thinking about, 177
  as problems separate from people,
    127–34, 148, 149
  strengths as exceptions to, 139–40
  Vision Statement and, *87*, 104
  working with, 74–76, 97
O'Byrne, Patrick, 25
office-based work, 153–55, 175
openness to help, 3–4, *62*, 63–64, *67*
organizational practices, 177–90
  ABC core principles and, 183–84
  climate and culture of, 190–99
  clinical discussion formats and, 187–90
  Collaborative Helping maps and, 69–90,
    177–83, 202
  collaborative spirit and, 192–97, 202
  paperwork and, 183–85
  staff and program evaluation and,
    185–97
  supervision and, 177–83, 198–99
organizing vision statement, 53, *54*, 55–58,
  71–74
  components of, 55–58, *67*
orienting questions, 44
Outcome Rating Scale (ORS), 186–87
outreach workers. *See* community-based
    work; helping workers; home-based
    work
over-responsible/under-responsible pattern,
  133–34, *134*, 136

paperwork, 183–85, 191
Parker, Sonja, 82, 88, 105–8
  Future House visual tool, 105–8, *106*
participation, sense of, 201

partner parents. *See* family partner
partnership, 30–31, 45, 200
Parton, Nigel, 25
passiveness, 110
Peck, C. J., 20
perpetual crises, 118, 119–20, 201
personal agency, 63, 148, 162
personality traits, 27
personal responsibility. *See* responsibility
personal stories, 7, 13, 129–30, 148,
    168–69
  private stories vs., 169
  See also life stories
physical abuse, 81, 88, 103–4, 109
  "No Problem Stance" and, 109–10,
    111, *111*
  See also Harm Statement; Safety
    Statement
plan
  for change, 112, 114–15, 116, 118
  Collaborative Helping maps and, 51,
    51, 64–67, *65, 67, 72, 87, 96*, 97,
    114–15, *169*, 181
  exception and, 114–15, 116, 118
Platinum Rule, 125
positives, focus on, 100–101, 104–5
possibilities
  believing in, 29–30, 200
  focus on, 53–54, 97, 102
power dynamics, 162–66
practical changes, 11
practice-based evidence, 17, 197
preconceived notions, 3
preference questions, 136, 149n4
preferred response questions, 136–37
pride, parental stories of, 101
Prison Mode, 82
private vs. personal stories., 169
proactive vision, 55
  Collaborative Helping maps and, 95
  coping strategies and, 127
  definition of, 102
  engagement and, 102–23
  plan for, 64, *65*
  possibilities focus of, 97
problematic situations, 134, 146–47
problems
  acknowledgment of, 102
  constraints focus and, 50

denial of, 109–10, *110*, 111
externalizing of, 59–61, 97,
    127–39, *135*
framing process for, 73–74
lack of control over, 109, 110–11, *111*
life goals and, 50–51
life story context of, 39
possibilities focus on, 53–54, 97, 102
questions about effects of, 136
recasting as obstacles, 97, 127–34
rethinking of, 125–49, 201
as separate from people, 74, 86–87, 97,
    127–34, 148, 201
separating self from, 127, 201
solution focus for, 61
problem-solving approach, 20
professional boundaries, 153–56, 162–75
  family partners and, 167–73
  more flexible definition of, 155–56, 175
  power dynamics and, 162–66
  principle-based approach to, 154
  traditional approaches and, 166–75, 175
professional ethics, 175
professional expertise, 195
professional privilege, 164–65
"professional speak," 165
program evaluation, 185, 186–87
psychotherapy, 26
Pulleyblank Coffey, Ellen, 49
purpose
  alignment of, 97
  clarification of, 178, *179*, 201
  sense of, 105
  spirituality and, 101

questions
  appreciative inquiry, 17, 104–5, 197–99
  assessment, 10
  change possibilities, 43–46, 139
  clinical discussion format, 188
  complaint to commitment, 104–5
  connection before correction, 113
  context of, 178
  corrective vs. facilitative, 44–46, 139
  externalizing, 132–33, 135–37
  facilitating intent, 44, 45–46, 139
  helpful, 42–43
  intentions, 143–44
  organizing vision, 56, 57–58, 64

orienting vs. influencing, 44
preference, 136, 149n4
preferred response, 136–37
Right Question Project, 173–74
scaling, 81, 89, 98n4, *106*, 107
strengths and supports, 142–44
"thought explorer," 40–41, 197
visioning, 105
See also inquiry

racial differences
    acknowledgment of, 5–6, 13
    supports from cultural values and,
        147–48
racism, 58, 134, 136
realistic goals, 56–57
recovery, formal definition of, 19
recovery-oriented models, 18–19, 49, 101
relational connection, 12–17, 20, 46–47,
        52–53, *62*, *67*, 97, 199, 201
    advocacy and, 173–74, 175
    to build desired futures, 123, 201
    building on supports and, 146–47
    before correction, 112, 113, 116, 117
    conversation and, 125
    how (process of), 12–14
    instances of, 100
    shifts in, 200
    what (content) of, 9–12
    why (purpose) of, 14–17
relational stance (attitude), 23, 26–33, 115
    family partner advocacy efforts and,
        161–62
    helping worker and, 199
relationship-based approach. *See*
        Collaborative Helping; helping
        workers
repetitive pattern, 146
residential programs
    ABCs of collaboration, 183–84, 194
    ABCs of staff evaluations, 185–86
    Collaborative Helping maps and, 69–78
    discharge from, 71–73
    family-centered, 77–78, 193–94
    overly restrictive placement in, 49
resilience, 18, 101, 202n2
resistance, 108
resourcefulness, 105, 107, 162
    eliciting, 29–33, 200

respect, 11, 27, 55
    organizing vision and, *54*, *67*
    shared desire for, 61
responsibility, 60, 148
    over/under pattern of, 133–34, *134*,
        136
Right Question Institute, 175n1
Right Question Project, 173–74
rituals, 37, 38
Rollnick, S., 17, 108
Root, E. A., 80, 103
Rothstein, Dan R., 173–74
Russell, S., 38, 127

safety
    actions in progress for, 88–89
    future actions for, 89
    Future House path of, 105–8, *106*
    goals setting for, 83, 87, 88, 90
    network of, 90
    parental discipline methods and, 103–4
    scaling questions about, 81, 89, 98n4
    signs of, 17, 196
Safety Plan, 83, 87, 88–91
Samuel, M., 190
Santana, Luz, 173–74
Saran Wrap, 131, 136
Sawyer, Tom (fictional), 93
scaling questions
    danger and safety, 81, 89, 98n4
    safety path visual representation of,
        106, 107
    supervisory Collaborative Helping
        Map, 180
Schoenwald, S. K., 17–18, 193
Screwed-up Belief, 132–33, 136, 138
self
    advocacy for, 173–74
    belief in, 7–8
    experiences of, 45–46, 64, 127
    sense of (*see* identity)
    separating from problem of, 127, 201
    use of, 39
self-blame, 74–75, 138
self-care, commitment to, 145–46
self-efficacy, 108, 116
self-harm, 119
self-marginalization, 164
self-stigmatization, 37

sense of self. *See* identity
separation, 52–56, 61–67, *67*
Session Rating Scale (SRS), 186, 187
sexism, 58
shame. *See* blame and shame
shared focus, 151
　forward-thinking vision and, 125
　lack of, 55
Sheinberg, Marcia, 101
Sheridan, K., 193
signs of safety approach, 17, 196
similarities, 13
Simon, Paul, 25
SMART format, 186
Sobell, L., 40
sociocultural context,
　acknowledgement of differences and,
　　5–6, 13
　building supports in, 147–48
　curiosity and, 2–3, 27–29, 200
　expectations and, 58, 61–62, *67*
　externalizing and, 138–39
　hopelessness and, 76
　parent-child relations and, 61–62, 63,
　　74–75
　placing problems in, 149n2
　responsiveness to, 2–6, 175
　story metaphor and, 35–37
solution-focused approaches, 51, 56–57,
　　102, 107
　child-protective work and, 17, 196
　solution-forced vs., 198
　specific relationship types and, 108–9
songs, 33–34
Sorensen, P. F., 17
Sparks, Jackie, 26, 186
spirituality, 101
staff evaluations, 185–87
statutory authority, 79
stereotypes, 13, 126
sticky messages, 55–56
stories. *See* life stories
story metaphor, 34–37, *34*, 46–47
　usefulness of, 35–37
strengths
　abstract concept of, 126
　acknowledging, 101
　conversations about, 142–49, 201
　as intentional practices, 139–44, 148, 149

recasting of, 74
rethinking of, 125, 126–27, 139–44,
　148–49
strengths-based approaches, 61, 74, 100–
　101, 125–26, 166, 196–97
substance misuse, 95, 109, 119, 145–46
　No Control Stance, 111
　No Problem Stance, 109–10, 111
　professional boundaries and, 156–57
　See also alcohol abuse
Summers, J. A., 187
supervision, 177–83, 202
　group, 198–99
Supervisory Collaborative Helping Map,
　177–83
　Agreed-Upon Focus, *179*, 180
　Introduction of the Person or Family,
　　178, *179*, 180
　Outline, *178*
　Purpose and Context, 178, *179*
　Reflection on Conversation, *179*, 180,
　　181
supportive help, 20, 139–40, 143, 154–55
supports, 139, 144, 145–46, 201
　Collaborative Helping maps, 200
　drawing on, 125
　identifying, 9, 51, *51*, 58–59, *62*,
　　63–64, *67*, *72*, 74
　informal Collaborative Helping Map,
　　92, *96*, 97
　new ways of thinking about, 177
　questions in conversations about,
　　142–44
　recasting of, 97
　on relational level, 146–47, 149
　at sociocultural level, 147–48
　supervisory Collaborative Helping Map,
　　179, 180, *180*
　vision statement and, *87*
　working with, 74–76
sympathy, expression of, 108
symptom reduction, shift from, 18, 101

taking the first step, 117–18
talking. *See* conversation; walking and
　talking
talk therapy, 8
team meetings, 198–99
therapeutic alliance, 26–27

therapy, 8, 195
  case management vs., 8
  outcomes of, 26
"thought explorer," 40–41, 197
time-outs, 89
Tomm, Karl, 44, 45, 60, 139, 149n3
trust, 55
  earning of, 3–4, 13, 201
  organizing vision and, *54, 67*
  shared desire for, 61
Trust-Go-Round, 147
Turnell, Andrew, 17, 26–27, 29–30, 54,
    82, 196
Twain, Mark, 93

unconscious motives, 195
urgency, sense of, 191, 192
U.S. Department of Health and Human
    Services, 18, 19, 101
U.S. Department of Labor, 21

validation, 11
values, 142, 143, 147–48, 149, 175, 201
VanDenBerg, J., 49
violence, 91, 109
vision of life's direction, 51, 64,
    102–23, 201
  agreed upon focus for, 126
  Child Protective Services and, 80–81,
    83, 102–8
  clarity of, 56
  Collaborative Helping maps and,
    83, 200
  discrepancy between current behavior
    and, 108
  engaging people toward, 102–23
  forward-thinking and, 53, 125
  Future House and, 105–8, *106,* 123n1
  goals and, 50, 51, 53–58, 108
  inspiration and, 97
  new ways of thinking about, 177
  organizing of, 53–58, *54, 67,* 71–74, *72*
  perpetual crises and, 118, 119–23, 201
  pessimism and, 104, 115–16,
    120–23, 140

  positive steps and, 145–46
  strengths as intentional practices and,
    139–44
  supports for, 144, 145–46
Vision Statement, 83–86, *87,* 90,
    102–3
  Child Protection Services context and,
    80–81, 102–4
  Safety Plan and, 83, 91
visitor relationships, 108, 109
Vogel, John, 202n1

Walker, W. S., 18
walking and talking, 8–9, 10, 37, 39,
    174–75
  guiding metaphor for, 151, 174
  helping interactions and, 118
  meaning of, 9, 151, 201–2
  residential treatment and, 75, 76
Walnum, Ellen, 159, 169, 175
Walsh, Froma, 101
Walsh, J., 20
Wambold, B. E., 26
"what is"/"what might be"/"what will
    be," 104
White, Michael, 17, 35, 38, 59, 127, 138,
    149n4
Whitney, D., 17
Winslade, J., 127
witnessing practices, 38
workloads, 191
work teams, 197–99
worry, 61–62, *62,* 63, *67,* 128, 133–34,
    136
Worrying Thoughts, 128–29
wraparound systems of care, 18, 19,
    49, 99
  approach of, 195–96
  family partners and, 159–62,
    167–73, 175
  organizational culture support for, 196

Yaeger, T. F., 17

Zimmerman, J. L., 127